A CARNIVORE'S DILEMMAS

AN UNAPOLOGETIC GUIDE TO NAVIGATING THE CHALLENGES OF A MEAT-FIRST LIFESTYLE

ZHAMEESHA LLC
ATLANTIS, FL (USA)

A Carnivore's Dilemmas
An Unapologetic Guide to Navigating the Challenges of a Meat-First Lifestyle

Copyright © 2025 by Stuart Barry Malin

ISBN 978-1-951645-26-7
First Edition, Print on Demand
Most recently updated 2026-02-26

Published by Zhameesha LLC
Atlantis, Florida USA
https://www.zhameesha.com

This book is a work of compassion.

BISAC Subject Headings (www.bisg.org)
HEA048000   HEALTH & FITNESS / Diet & Nutrition / General
SEL000000   SELF-HELP / General
POL000000   POLITICAL SCIENCE / General

12 11 10 9 8 7 6 5 4 3 2 1

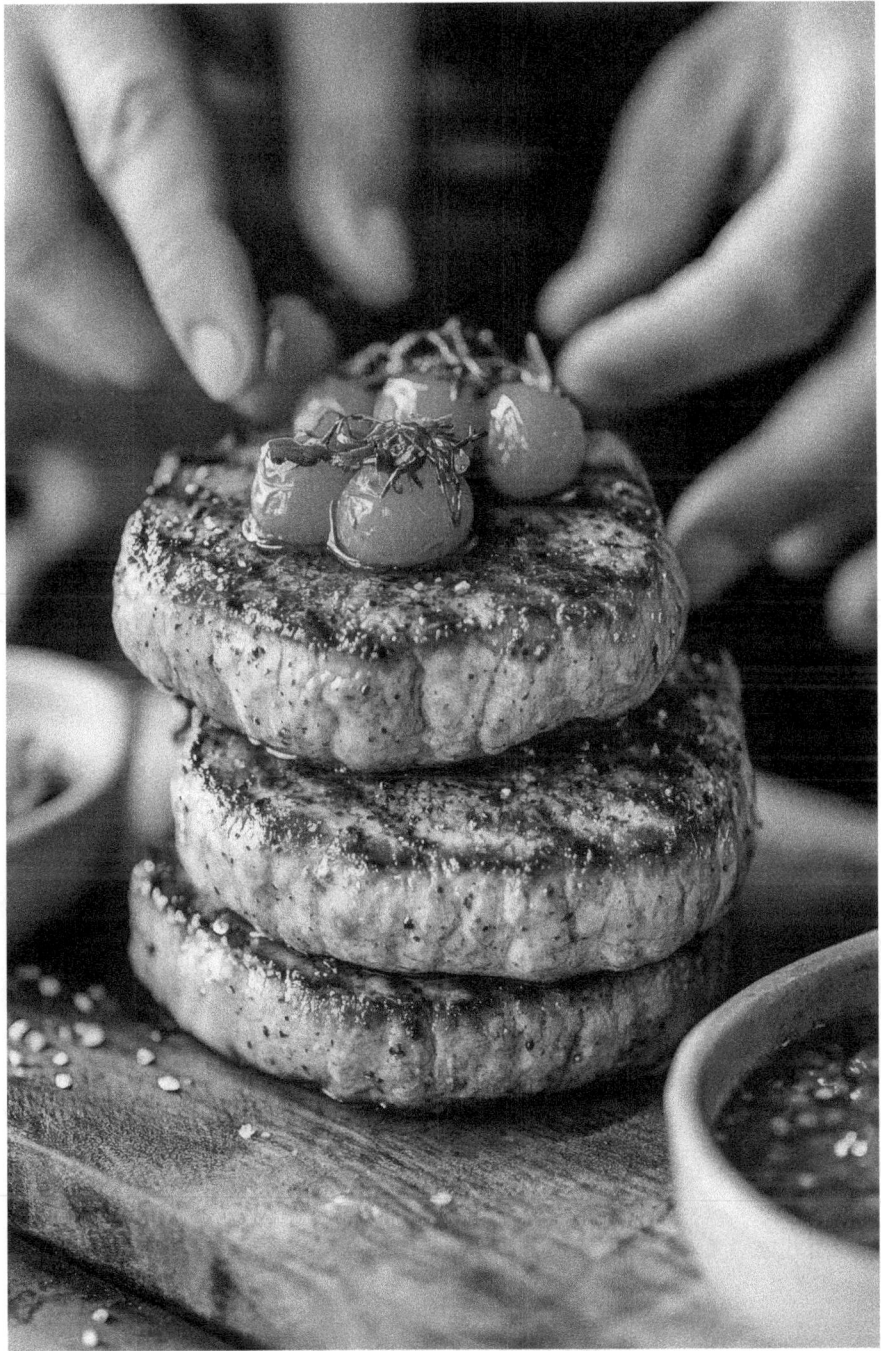

Welcome to **A Carnivore's Dilemmas**. This book isn't about rules or dogma; it's about the navigating the challenges of real situations in a world where embracing a meat-first lifestyle can feel as isolating as it is empowering.

For me, this journey began with the need to isolate and eliminate food sensitivities and grew into a way of life. Like many, I've faced doubts, struggles, and plenty of awkward conversations. But I've also discovered a path that's transformed how I feel, think, and live.

In these pages, I'll share a collection of dilemmas—personal, practical, and sometimes philosophical—that arise when we choose to eat differently than the majority. These dilemmas aren't just theoretical; they've shown up in my life and in the lives of others I've connected with on this path. From navigating social situations to grappling with deeply held beliefs about food and health, this book reflects the real-world questions we face as carnivores.

Whether you're just starting to explore this lifestyle or you've been on this path for years, my hope is that these stories and insights will resonate with you. I hope they'll spark ideas, provide clarity, and, most importantly, remind you that you're not alone on this journey.

This book is an invitation—to reflect, to experiment, and to embrace the joys and challenges of choosing a path less traveled. It's about finding your own way forward with confidence and authenticity.

Welcome to *A Carnivore's Dilemma*. I'm so glad you're here.

About this Book

This book expresses my experiences and point-of-view

The content os this book is derived from my own journey as I zig-zag a path that enables me to embrace the Carnivore lifestyle.

- The *situations* are not fabricated but come from reflection on real life and from notes taken while out-and-about in the world.
- The *assessments* are made in a context of much research undertaken over many months to better understand Carnivore by listening to a number of health practitioners and meat-first advocates on **YouTube**.
- The *counsel* offered comes from discussions about the situations and the consideration in the context of available information, all biased in favor of a meat-based diet.
- The *sources* of this information are varied and compellingly argue against the consumption of plant-based foods.

This book was produced with the assistance of AI

For this book, I worked with OpenAI's ChatGTP o3 model.

- I engaged in conversations with the ChatGTP to explore topics and situations of my selection.
- Most of the text of the sections were generated by the ChatGTP.
- I reviewed, edited, and reformatted all of the text

The perspectives presented are authentically my own.

Disclaimer and a call for caution

I believe that a carnivore diet is better *for me*. It <u>may</u> offer potential benefits *for you*. My experience confirms the potential for reducing inflammation, improving metabolic health, and optimizing nutrient intake. However, as is often said, "your mileage may vary."

I am not a health practitioners and do not offer this book as medical advice. The following points cannot be understated:

- The importance of developing a personal response relevant to your life situations.
- Giving mindful attention to potential illness considerations and/or nutrient deficiencies
- Developing a personal approach to adopting and maintaining a dietary practice, especially one as rigorous as Carnivore.

More rigorous scientific research is needed to fully understand the long-term effects and potential risks and benefits of a carnivore diet. My journey so far has been relatively short term.

Consult with your Physician

- *It is important to consult with a healthcare professional before making any significant dietary changes, especially if you have pre-existing health conditions or are taking medications.*

- *The information presented here must not be considered medical advice.*

- *Consulting with qualified healthcare professionals is crucial for personalized guidance.*

How best to engage the content

You can peruse this book in any order that strikes you, including opening randomly, for, as you will find explored in various arenas and on some of the pages, the notion of "entanglement" is a compelling counter-argument to truly random

I (Stuart, a human) once asked Pi (an AI collaborator of mine), "Can you explain 'entanglement' in a spiritual sense."
Here is what Pi replied with:

> *In a spiritual sense, entanglement refers to the idea that everything in the universe, including living beings, is connected on a deeper, invisible level. This concept goes beyond the physical connections we can observe and suggests that there is an underlying unity that binds all things together.*
>
> *Entanglement in a spiritual context implies that our thoughts, emotions, and actions can influence and be influenced by the world around us in ways that might not be immediately obvious. It's often associated with ideas like synchronicity, karma, and the interconnectedness of all living things.*
>
> *The notion of spiritual entanglement encourages us to consider the impact of our choices on the world and on others, and to recognize that we are all part of a larger, interconnected whole.*

Death is not an option, but Life is

If you don't choose Life,

You'll get a laborious ride to death,

Which will come perhaps as a welcomed exit.

It is my belief that to choose Carnivore is to choose Life.

Publisher's Note (February 2026)

When this book was first written, it stood on its own—an honest record of inquiry, experience, and understanding at a particular moment in time.

Since then, additional books have emerged from the same lived investigation into animal-based nutrition. Taken together, they now form what the author has come to recognize as **The Carnivore Continuum**: an evolving, experience-driven exploration of carnivore eating as it is actually practiced, questioned, challenged, and integrated over time.

This volume represents one position along that continuum. It reflects what was known, tested, and understood when it was written—and remains unchanged for that reason. Readers may encounter perspectives elsewhere in the series that refine, complicate, or extend what appears here. That is intentional.

The Continuum is not a doctrine.
It is a record of attention.

Contents

Welcome

Welcome to A Carnivore's Dilemmas i

About this Book ii

Disclaimer and a call for caution iii

Consult with your Physician iv

How best to engage the content v

Death is not an option, but Life is vi

Publisher's Note vii

Introduction

About this Carnivore 3

Why This Book Exists 5

The Grand Dilemma 6

What This Book Is (and Isn't) 9

An Invitation 10

The Dilemmas — Dietary Intake

Is It Okay to Eat Some Plant-Based or Plant-Derived Foods? 15

Poultry 19

Indulgences 23

Meat Choices 27

Alcohol: Beer, wine, liquor 31

Sugar – Be Careful! 37

Meat and Potatoes: Is That Really So Bad? 41

The Dilemmas — Social Consequences

The Sustainability and Ethics of Meat Consumption 45

If Plants Are Genuinely Toxic, Why Are They So Prevalent in Human Diets? 49

People Will Tell You That Your Diet Is Unhealthy 54

Be Careful with Your Assertiveness 57

A Loss of Interest in Romantic Partners Who Are Plant-Eaters 61

Going to Social Outings Where Food Is Central 64

Do You Try to Convince Others to Take on Carnivore? 68

On Vegetarians: Navigating Differences with Grace 73

People Will Tell You That You Are Too Thin 77

The Dilemmas — Being Carnivore

The Personal Journey of Being Carnivore 83

Leadership and Partnership in the Carnivore Journey 86

Attitudes About Hygiene May Change, Radically 89

A Feeling of Revoltingness at Plants-as-Food 92

How Restrictive Should I Be? 95

Blood Work: Expect Changes 99

Supplements - Fewer are needed 104

Has it gotten warmer? 108

As a Carnivore, You Are Not Representative of "Normal" 112

Tracking Your Progress 115

N=1 Science: The Call of Personal Experimentation 119

Transgressions Become More Painful 120

A Small Bit of Metabolic Science

Overview of Glucose Metabolism 127

Overview of Fat Metabolism 131

Overview of Carbohydrate Metabolism 135

Overview of Calories 139

Overview of Cholesterol 143

Overview of Ketones and Ketosis 146

Ketogenesis in a Meat-Centric Diet 150

Postmatter

About The Author 157

Points of Contact 159

The Carnivore Continuum 160

This book is a meal that will nourish you! 161

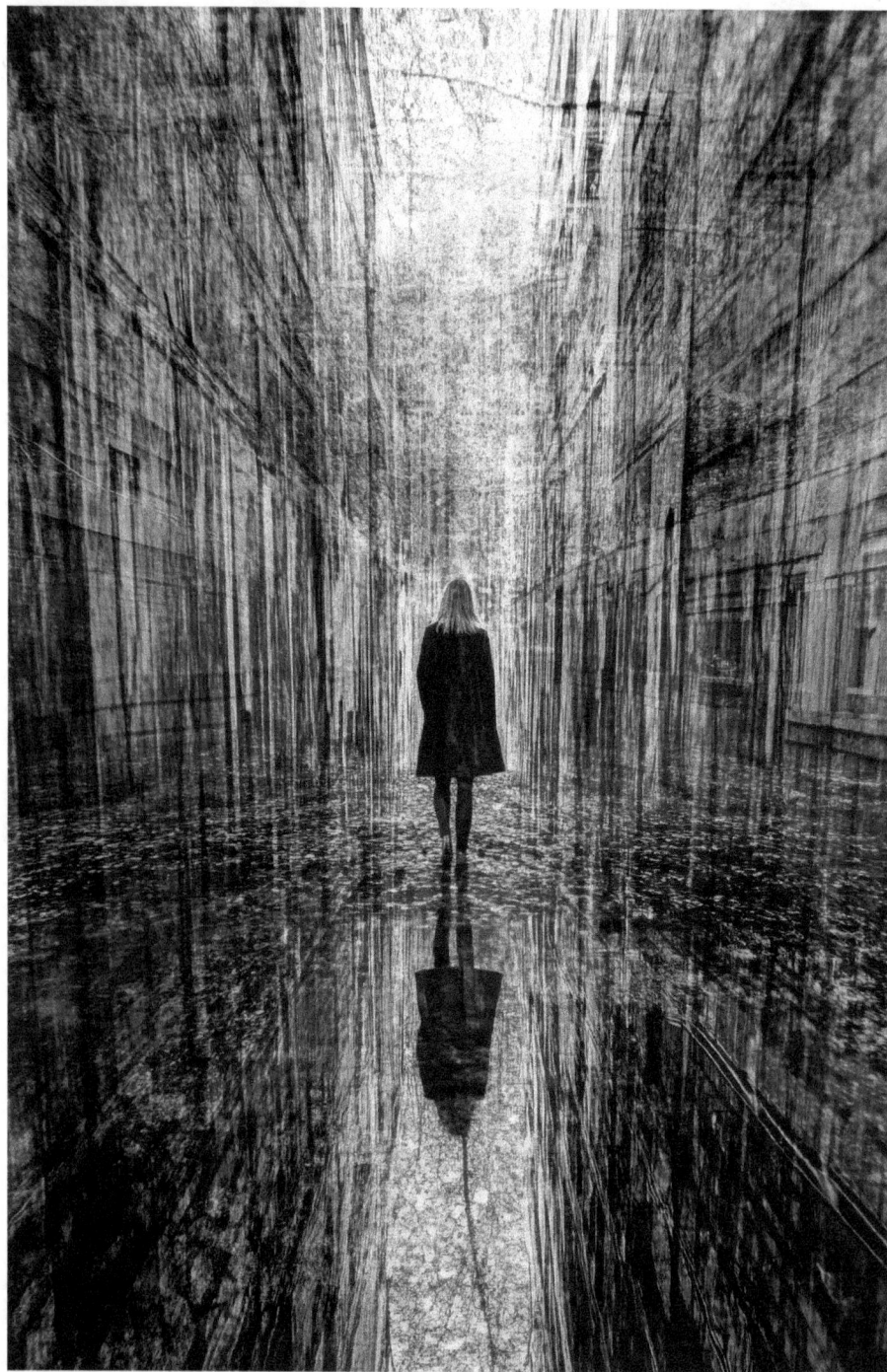

INTRODUCTION

About this Carnivore

I started down the path toward Carnivore without intending to be "a Carnivore" or even knowing about Carnivore as a dietary lifestyle. I was led to Carnivore by the need to eliminate ear more "foods" in search of what was causing me frequent headaches and debilitating brain fog. The more I eliminated, the better I felt, but then would reintroduce the offenders in a search for the one culprit. Little did I imagine that the culprit was as widespread as plants.

I have long been into health and am an invertebrate supplementer, especially exploring the esoteric substances with purported benefits for longevity and health span. These are the subject of some future book. What matters now, for this introduction, is that I have long been averse to sugars and carbs, and have attempted to be "keto" (but was doing so with a dominantly plant-based approach.

A good number of years ago, I identified wheat as a trigger for terrible brain fog events. Over time, I discovered this was the case in America, but that I could consume bread without such impact when in southern Europe. This led to a hypothesis that the impact could be from the increasing use of Glyphosate, even as a drying agent.

My greatest surprise was when I identified arugula as a trigger of brain fog. Investigation on YouTube led me deep into the Carnivore community, and from the teachings, perspectives, guidance, and stories I encountered there, I increased my meat consumption.

This was a somewhat radical step for me as though I had been eating meat, and did so in my teens, the years in between saw me take on vegetarianism and even a few years as a raw foodist. In hindsight, these were my most unhealthy times.

As of the time of this writing, I have been mostly "hardcore" Carnivore for about nine months. Yes, less than a year, and I feel so vibrant. I have lost about 20 pounds (going from 180 to 160, at six foot one inch). I am very pleased with the transformation of my body composition.

I "conduct" many personal experiments with what I eat, including indulgences (oh, I so love ice cream when I am in Spain but avoid it in America), and transgressions (for fabulous ethnic food experiences when traveling, especially in London). These and other experiences constitute the core of the themes and dilemmas discussed in this book.

I am fortunate that my writing colleague, Andrew Wallis — see our fabulous fiction series on Amazon (The Epic of The OAI) or at www.TheOAI.com — has embraced this journey of restrictive eating with me. It makes eating a meal more pleasant to have someone who is satisfied with a high-fat meal and will shun the transgressions.

I am also fortunate that my mother, who lives nearby to me and who I see weekly for a meal (lunch or dinner), is quite happy with a meat-only of meat-dominated meal. We both adore great BBQ.

I am fortunate also for the great diversity of high quality animal products available to me, such as at/from Wild Fork and Whole Foods.

Why This Book Exists

This book exists because I am on the journey and have experiences that may be of benefit to others.

As a writer, I can organize my thoughts and and can present them. As an advocate of collaborating with AI, I can perform research and organize material with rapidity.

Further, in the spirit of speed and collaboration with AI, I reframe much of my thinking and writing through the writing of the AI. For this book, I have worked with ChatGTP. This chapter, and the preceding one, are written entirely by me.

I offer this book to "you" not to advocate that you take up Carnivore — that is a crucial and personal decision — but if you choose to do so, to gain insight or other benefit from my experiences.

I have another book on Amazon regarding the meat-first lifestyle which was generated by having AI assist me to digest, organize, and present key ideas of Carnivore from leaders in the community. The sources for this were videos on YouTube. I hope this book can help people interested in the Carnivore diet/lifestyle to better understand it. Please look for it: ***Carnivore: What, Why, How***

The Grand Dilemma

"The Grand Dilemma" encapsulates the overarching challenge of adopting and sustaining a meat-first lifestyle in a modern world that is not only tailored for but actively reinforces plant-based and mixed-diet norms. It is the convergence of countless smaller dilemmas—personal, social, cultural, and scientific—that together create a larger, more profound question:

How do we align our dietary choices with our values, goals, and biological needs while navigating a world that often resists, misunderstands, or actively opposes them?

Core Aspects of the Grand Dilemma

1.   *Cultural and Social Norms*

- Most societies have embraced plant-based or mixed diets as the default.
- Navigating social situations, relationships, and cultural traditions that center around carb-heavy or plant-dominant meals can be isolating or alienating.

2.   *Medical and Scientific Skepticism*

- Medical norms and dietary guidelines are built on research that primarily reflects mixed or plant-based populations.
- Carnivore markers often fall outside the "normal" ranges, leading to unnecessary alarm or pushback from healthcare providers.

3.   *Economic and Environmental Criticisms*

- The meat-first lifestyle is often portrayed as unsustainable or environmentally harmful, despite compelling counterarguments about regenerative agriculture and the ecological role of ruminants.

- Carnivores are often accused of ethical or environmental irresponsibility, making it difficult to advocate for this lifestyle without facing resistance.

4.   *The Personal Journey*

- As Carnivores, we face a continuous cycle of self-experimentation and adaptation to find what works for our bodies.

- Personal dilemmas, such as cravings, convenience, and long-term sustainability, add complexity to the lifestyle.

5.   *The Philosophical Tension*

Carnivores often challenge prevailing worldviews, not just about food but about health, ethics, and the nature of human civilization. This can lead to a profound sense of alignment — or alienation — from the larger society.

The Heart of the Grand Dilemma

At its core, the *Grand Dilemma* is about balancing authenticity and practicality:

- *Authenticity* to pursue a lifestyle that feels aligned with your health, values, and experiences.

- *Practicality* to exist harmoniously within a world that operates by different rules and expectations.

You are your Best Champion

"N=1" refers to experiments conducted on a single subject—you. Unlike traditional scientific studies that analyze data from large groups, N=1 experiments focus on personal observations and outcomes, recognizing that what works for one person may not work for another.

N=1 science empowers you to discover what truly works for your body.

- Personal experimentation allows you to build a unique, sustainable, and effective approach to the Carnivore lifestyle.
- It's a practice of curiosity, commitment, and self-leadership—core aspects of thriving in the face of the Grand Dilemma.

Freedom = Responsibility

The **Grand Dilemma** is the freedom and necessity to find what is true and works for you.

- *The Grand Dilemma* is not just a question of what we eat—it's a question of how we live.
- *The Grand Dilemma* is a journey of self-discovery and resilience, where every individual Carnivore must navigate the crossroads of science, tradition, and personal conviction while crafting their unique path.

What This Book Is (and Isn't)

This book is a candid exploration of real-world challenges and thoughtful ways about how they may be addressed.

This book is <u>not</u> a *how-to manual* nor is it a defense of carnivory.

The dilemmas I present are personal. You may or may not experience the situations or find them a conundrum.

I offer an unapologetic perspective on them. By unapologetic, I mean that there's no discussion to be had now, and, I am free to change my perspective in the future!

I hope that my explorations of these situations provides you with insights, and you take away practical strategies whether you are curious about or committed to the carnivore lifestyle.

An Invitation

This book is an exploration of the challenges, insights, and unexpected joys that come with stepping outside the norm to embrace a meat-first lifestyle. It's a journey into questions that may already resonate with you and perhaps ones you've yet to consider.

Please approach the dilemmas with an open mind, ready to explore your own carnivore journey.

As you dive into this collection of dilemmas, here's what I invite you to take away:

1.   *A Deeper Understanding of Yourself*

Discover how a carnivore lifestyle reshapes your body, your energy, and even your relationship with food. You'll come to see how these changes reflect broader transformations in your life.

2.   *Practical Tools for Navigating Challenges*

Whether it's dealing with social situations, decoding metabolic science, or managing setbacks, this book offers real-world insights to help you confidently navigate the road ahead.

3.   *Empowerment Through Awareness*

Learn to separate fact from fiction, to challenge assumptions about health and nutrition, and to rely on your own experiences rather than conventional norms.

4.   *A Connection to a Like-Minded Community*

Recognize that you're not alone in questioning the status quo. The dilemmas explored here are shared by many, and through this book, you'll find camaraderie in those who walk this unconventional path.

5.   *A New Perspective on Food and Health*

Shift your focus from fitting into "normal" to understanding what truly works for you. Embrace the clarity and simplicity that comes from aligning your diet with your body's needs.

This book is both personal and universal. While it reflects my journey and perspective, it's written for anyone who is navigating their own carnivore path. Take what resonates, explore what challenges you, and trust yourself to find what fits.

> *Above all, this is an invitation to reflect, adapt, and thrive.*
> *Thank you for joining me on this journey. Let's embrace the*
> *dilemmas together and uncover what lies on the other side.*

THE DILEMMAS
DIETARY INTAKE

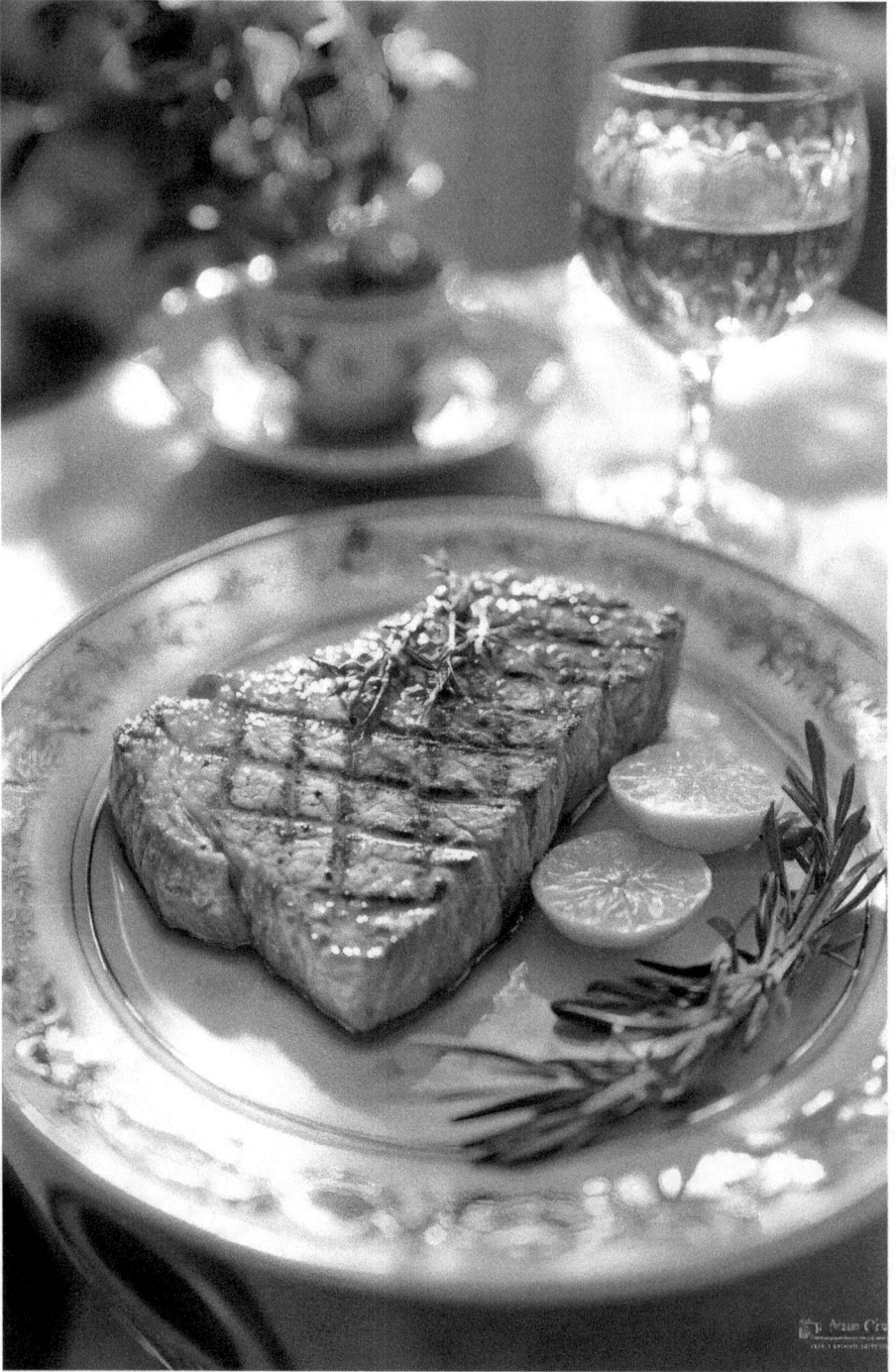

Is It Okay to Eat Some Plant-Based or Plant-Derived Foods?

For many who adopt the carnivore diet, the initial question of whether plants can or should be part of their meals is both practical and philosophical. While the fundamental premise of the carnivore lifestyle emphasizes the potential harms of consuming plants—citing antinutrients, toxins, and their historical role as survival food rather than optimal nourishment—societal norms, personal habits, and social settings often complicate this principle.

1. Plants as Survival Food, Not Optimal Nourishment

Throughout history, plants have served as fallback food in times of scarcity. This perspective reframes plants not as the cornerstone of a healthy diet but as something humans consumed to survive when more nutrient-dense animal foods were unavailable. Modern science bolsters this view, revealing that many plants contain compounds (e.g., oxalates, lectins, phytates) that can irritate the gut, disrupt nutrient absorption, or trigger inflammatory responses.

For those transitioning to a carnivore lifestyle, this understanding can lead to a growing reluctance to consume plants, particularly as they notice adverse effects, such as:

- *Digestive discomfort:* Bloating, cramping, or irregular bowel movements.
- *Mental effects:* Brain fog or mood instability.
- *Physical symptoms:* Fatigue, joint pain, or inflammatory responses.

2. The Role of Habit and Social Expectations

Despite this accumulating evidence, many carnivores find themselves grappling with habits, preferences, and cultural norms shaped by a lifetime of plant consumption. Plant-based foods often hold sentimental value (childhood meals, favorite dishes) or serve as the centerpiece of social events and gatherings. In restaurants, menus are designed with plants as either the main feature or essential accompaniment to meat-based dishes.

3. The Evolution of Tolerance and Taste

A fascinating phenomenon for many carnivores is how their taste for plants diminishes over time. What once seemed essential—salads, side dishes, desserts—becomes increasingly unappealing as they attune their palates to the simplicity and satisfaction of meat. Simultaneously, the physical and mental disruptions caused by plant foods become more pronounced, fostering an intuitive aversion.

4. Navigating "Transgressions"

For those who occasionally consume plant-based or plant-derived foods, the results often reinforce their commitment to carnivore principles. Whether it's a deliberate indulgence or a necessity in social settings, the aftermath—digestive upset, mental fog, or general discomfort—acts as a reminder of why they chose this path.

Practical Strategies for Addressing the Question

1.   Define Your Boundaries

Every individual's journey is unique. For some, complete abstinence from plants is the ideal. Others may allow limited exceptions—like herbs, spices, or occasional indulgences—while still adhering to the core principles of a meat-first lifestyle.

2.   Social and Cultural Adaptations

In situations where avoiding plants entirely is difficult, focus on minimizing their presence and prioritizing the most nutrient-dense foods available. For example:

- Choose dishes where meat is the primary component, even if it's paired with vegetables.
- Politely decline sides or request substitutions when dining out.
- At social gatherings, eat beforehand or bring your own carnivore-friendly options.

3.   Listen to Your Body

Ultimately, the strongest guide is your own experience. Over time, the physical and mental signals your body provides after consuming plants will clarify what works for you and what doesn't.

4.   Cultivate Understanding

Recognize that your evolving aversion to plant foods is part of the broader transformation of identity, relationships, and perceptions. It's not simply about "following the rules" but about aligning with what makes you feel healthiest and most authentic.

The Larger Dilemma

The question of eating plants reflects a central tension of the carnivore lifestyle: living authentically in a world designed for a very different paradigm. While society celebrates plant-based diets as moral, sustainable, and healthful, carnivores challenge this narrative through their lived experiences. Over time, this question evolves from one of permissibility to one of preference and principle, as individuals align their choices with their growing awareness of what truly nourishes their bodies and minds.

Poultry

Poultry occupies an interesting and somewhat ambivalent position within the carnivore diet. For many, it serves as a transition food—a stepping stone for those hesitant to fully embrace red meat and other nutrient-dense animal products. Yet, for committed carnivores, poultry often feels less satisfying, raising questions about its role in a meat-centric lifestyle.

Poultry as a Transition Food

1.   Familiarity and Acceptance

Chicken and turkey are often the most socially accepted forms of animal protein, appealing to individuals who are cautious about consuming red meat. These meats are considered "safe" or "light" options, making them a common choice for those newly exploring an animal-based diet.

2.   Preference for Low-Fat Cuts

Many people opt for lean cuts like chicken breast, avoiding the more nutrient-rich, higher-fat portions. This preference reflects broader societal norms about low-fat eating, which may not align with the carnivore philosophy of prioritizing fats for energy and nutrition.

The Limitations of Poultry

1.   Nutritional Simplicity

Compared to red meats like beef and lamb, poultry is nutritionally less dense. While it provides protein, it lacks the abundance of vitamins, minerals, and fatty acids that make red meat a cornerstone of the carnivore diet.

2.   Taste and Satisfaction

Many carnivores find that as their palate adapts to the richness of red meat, poultry becomes less appealing. The taste is often described as bland or one-dimensional, leading to a sense of dissatisfaction when consumed as a primary food source.

Maximizing the Benefits of Poultry

1.   Choose Fatty Cuts

If you include poultry in your diet, prioritize the darker, fattier parts, such as thighs, drumsticks, and skin. These cuts are more flavorful and provide the fats necessary for energy and satiation in a carnivore diet.

2.   Whole Animal Consumption

Eating the entire bird, including organ meats, can enhance the nutritional profile of poultry. The liver, heart, and other parts offer valuable nutrients that are often overlooked when consuming only lean muscle meat.

The Challenges of Modern Poultry Production

1.   Industrial Farming Practices

In the United States, much of the poultry available in supermarkets is the product of industrial-scale farming. Modern chickens and turkeys have been selectively bred to grow quickly and yield more meat, often at the expense of nutritional quality.

2.   Diet and Conditions

Poultry raised on unnatural diets of grains and soy lacks the nutritional benefits of animals raised on traditional, species-appropriate foods like insects. These feeding practices, combined with confined living conditions, result in meat that is less nutrient-dense and potentially laden with residues from antibiotics and hormones.

Sourcing High-Quality Poultry

1.   Seek Traditional Practices

For those who choose to include poultry, it's worth investing in animals raised on natural diets. Chickens and turkeys allowed to forage for bugs and other natural foods produce meat with a better nutrient profile and superior taste.

2.   Support Local Producers

Buying poultry from small-scale or regenerative farms not only supports sustainable practices but also ensures you're consuming a product closer to what nature intended.

Poultry in Perspective

While poultry can play a role in a carnivore diet, it's unlikely to be the centerpiece for those seeking the fullest benefits of this lifestyle. It serves as a stepping stone for some and as an occasional addition for others. By understanding its limitations and making mindful choices about sourcing and preparation, poultry can complement a meat-first approach without compromising nutritional goals or satisfaction.

> *In the end, the role of poultry is a personal choice—one that reflects your individual preferences, priorities, and values within the broader framework of the carnivore diet.*

Indulgences

Indulgences occupy a unique space within the carnivore lifestyle, representing a conscious departure from strict dietary principles in favor of personal enjoyment. Whether these indulgences are rare holiday treats, everyday staples like coffee, or habit-forming pleasures such as chocolate, they introduce complexity and choice into an otherwise streamlined way of eating.

The Role of Indulgences

1.   Elective and Intentional Choices

Indulgences are inherently personal and optional. As long as they are consumed with awareness and intentionality, they can coexist within a carnivore framework. Recognizing them as deliberate choices—rather than lapses—empowers individuals to maintain control over their diet while allowing room for enjoyment.

2.   The Pleasure Principle

Many indulgences are plant-based or derived and are enjoyed for their psychoactive effects, such as caffeine in coffee, theobromine in chocolate, or sweetness in natural sweeteners like stevia and monk fruit. These compounds trigger pleasure responses, adding an element of joy to consumption.

Balancing Indulgence and Health

1.   Understanding the Consequences

While indulgences can provide temporary satisfaction, they often come with trade-offs. For some, they may introduce digestive discomfort, inflammation, or mental fogginess, which can detract from the benefits of a meat-based diet.

2.   Testing and Awareness

It can be helpful to periodically abstain from indulgences to better understand their effects. A brief withdrawal allows individuals to evaluate whether these items enhance or detract from their overall well-being.

3.   Mindful Integration

Rather than defaulting to indulgences as a routine part of life, consider setting boundaries around their frequency and quantity. This ensures they remain special and do not undermine the core principles of the carnivore lifestyle.

The Debate Among Carnivores

1.   The "Hardcore" Perspective

Some adherents of the carnivore diet advocate for complete abstinence from plant-derived foods and compounds, viewing them as toxins that conflict with the goals of the lifestyle. For these individuals, indulgences are seen as compromises that dilute the diet's purity and effectiveness.

2.   A Holistic View

Others take a more balanced approach, emphasizing that optimal health is not only about physical well-being but also about mental and emotional fulfillment. Occasional indulgences, enjoyed responsibly, can be part of a well-rounded and satisfying life.

Common Indulgences and Their Impacts

1.   Coffee and Tea

- Benefits: Provides energy, focus, and ritual.
- Potential Drawbacks: May cause jitters, dependency, or digestive issues.

2.   Chocolate

- Benefits: Rich flavor and pleasure-inducing compounds like theobromine.
- Potential Drawbacks: High in oxalates and can trigger cravings for sweets.

3.   Natural Sweeteners (Stevia, Monk Fruit)

- Benefits: Adds sweetness without spiking blood sugar.
- Potential Drawbacks: May perpetuate a desire for sweet flavors, making it harder to transition away from plant-derived foods.

4.   Holiday or Special Treats

- Benefits: Connects us to traditions and celebrations.
- Potential Drawbacks: Can derail dietary consistency if overindulged.

Indulgences in Perspective

Indulgences reflect the inherent balance between discipline and pleasure in the carnivore lifestyle. While the strictest adherents may see them as unnecessary or counterproductive, most carnivores understand that life is about more than rigid rules—it's about finding joy and meaning within one's choices.

By treating indulgences as intentional, conscious acts, you can enjoy them without guilt while staying aligned with your broader health goals. Whether you choose to abstain entirely or incorporate them sparingly, the key is understanding their role in your life and making informed decisions that resonate with your values and priorities.

Meat Choices

The carnivore diet offers a unique opportunity to explore the vast diversity of animal foods, both in terms of types of meat and preparation methods. It invites a departure from the conventional focus on muscle cuts and encourages a broader appreciation for the variety of nutrients and flavors animals can provide. By making thoughtful meat choices, one can maximize the health benefits of the diet while also supporting ethical and sustainable practices.

Exploring a Wide Variety of Meats

1.   Beyond Beef: Bison, Elk, and More

Carnivore encourages individuals to look beyond the supermarket staples of beef, chicken, and pork. Game meats such as bison, elk, venison, and even less common proteins like duck or rabbit can provide a richer nutritional profile and unique flavors. These meats are often leaner, and their wild or semi-wild upbringing typically ensures higher-quality fats and fewer artificial inputs.

2.   Organ Meats: Nature's Superfoods

Organs like liver, heart, kidney, and spleen are nutrient powerhouses packed with essential vitamins, minerals, and unique compounds that are hard to obtain from muscle meat alone. Incorporating these into your diet supports overall health and reflects the ancestral practice of consuming the "whole animal."

Prioritizing Meat Quality

1.   Grass-Fed and Pasture-Raised

Meat from grass-fed and pasture-raised animals is superior in fat quality, containing higher levels of omega-3 fatty acids, conjugated linoleic acid (CLA), and fat-soluble vitamins like A, D, E, and K. These animals are raised on diets more natural to their species, avoiding the potential harm caused by grain-based feeds.

2.   Wild-Caught and Heritage Breeds

Whenever possible, choose meats from wild-caught or heritage breeds, as these animals are typically more robust, healthier, and raised without the high-input systems of industrial farming.

3.   Avoid Feedlot-Meat When Possible

Animals raised on corn, soy, and other industrial feed not only produce lower-quality fats but also contribute to the industrial farming practices that many find objectionable. Shifting to higher-quality meat aligns with both health and ethical considerations.

Focusing on Fat Over Protein

1.   Why Fat Matters

Fat should be the primary macronutrient in a carnivore diet, providing energy, supporting hormonal health, and enhancing satiety. Carnivores are often advised to aim for at least 70-80% of their caloric intake from fat. This can be achieved by selecting fatty cuts of meat like ribeye, brisket, or pork belly, and incorporating supplemental fats like tallow, butter, or suet.

2.   Protein: A Supporting Role

While protein is crucial for maintaining muscle mass and bodily functions, consuming excessive protein can lead to gluconeogenesis, where the body converts excess protein into glucose. By focusing on fat as the main energy source, you ensure optimal metabolic health and energy efficiency.

Sustainable and Ethical Considerations

1.   Supporting Regenerative Farming

Choosing meat from farms practicing regenerative agriculture supports soil health, biodiversity, and carbon sequestration. This aligns with many carnivores' broader values of living in harmony with nature.

2.   Respecting the Animal

Eating nose-to-tail minimizes waste and honors the life of the animal. Using bones for broth, consuming organs, and even exploring delicacies like marrow or tongue enriches the diet while fostering a deeper connection to the food source.

Practical Tips for Meat Choices

1.   Stock Up on Staples

Keep your freezer well-stocked with essentials like fatty cuts of beef, ground meats, and organ meats. Having a variety ensures you never feel limited.

2.   Experiment with New Cuts and Preparations

Try slow-cooking brisket, grilling lamb chops, or searing duck breast to expand your culinary repertoire. Incorporating diversity keeps meals exciting and satisfying.

3.   Supplement Fat When Needed

If your meat is too lean, add fat through butter, ghee, or rendered animal fats. Avoid relying too heavily on lean meats like chicken breast or turkey, as they lack sufficient fat for energy needs.

Meat Choices as a Cornerstone of Carnivore

Your meat choices are central to the success and sustainability of the carnivore lifestyle. By embracing variety, prioritizing quality, and maintaining a focus on fat, you can ensure optimal health, satisfaction, and alignment with personal values. Exploring different types of meat and expanding beyond the basics is not only practical but also deeply rewarding, offering both nourishment and a deeper appreciation for the richness of animal-based eating.

Alcohol: Beer, wine, liquor

Alcoholic beverages hold a unique position in modern culture, straddling the lines between indulgence, social glue, and stress management. For many, they are inseparable from celebrations, gatherings, and personal rituals. While alcohol consumption is not inherently aligned with a carnivore lifestyle, it is ultimately a personal choice that balances individual goals, health priorities, and cultural habits.

Alcohol and the Carnivore Lifestyle

1.   Plant Origins

Most alcoholic beverages are plant-based or plant-derived. This may conflict with the foundational principles of a carnivore diet, which emphasizes avoiding plant toxins and anti-nutrients.

2.   Carbohydrate Content

Alcoholic beverages vary widely in carbohydrate content, potentially interfering with ketosis or metabolic processes optimized by a meat-centric diet.

Types of Alcoholic Beverages

Each category of alcohol presents different considerations for those on a carnivore diet:

1.   Beer

Derived from grains and typically brewed with hops, beer contains the most plant material.

Concerns:

- Gluten sensitivity: Many beers contain gluten, which can irritate those with sensitivities.
- Phytoestrogens: Hops contain compounds that mimic estrogen, potentially affecting hormonal balance, particularly in men.

Recommendation: If consuming beer, opt for gluten-free varieties and be mindful of quantity.

2.   Wine

Made from fermented grapes, wine is often considered a "better" alcohol choice due to its lower carbohydrate content (especially in dry varieties) and potential health benefits.

Potential Benefits:

- Polyphenols, such as resveratrol, may have antioxidant properties.
- Wine can be lower in carbohydrates than beer.

Concerns:

- Residual sugars in sweeter wines can add carbohydrates.
- Sulfites and additives may cause sensitivities in some individuals.

3.   Distilled Liquors (Spirits)

Distilled alcohols like whiskey, vodka, gin, and rum have minimal carbohydrates but deliver a high concentration of alcohol.

Considerations:

- Minimal plant residue due to distillation.
- Barrel aging introduces chemical compounds, such as tannins, which are not animal-derived.
- Mixing with sweetened beverages or syrups adds sugars.

Recommendation: Stick to straight liquors or mix with soda water to avoid additional carbohydrates.

4.   Sweetened Beverages and Cocktails

Many mixed drinks and flavored spirits contain sugars or syrups, compounding the impact of alcohol on blood sugar and metabolism.

Avoidance Tip: Opt for unsweetened mixers, such as soda water, or consume liquor neat.

The Metabolic Impact of Alcohol

1.   Alcohol as a Macronutrient

- Alcohol provides 7 calories per gram, nearly as energy-dense as fat (9 calories/gram).
- Unlike fat or protein, alcohol is metabolized first, potentially stalling fat-burning processes like ketosis.

2.   Effects on Hormones

- Beer's phytoestrogens from hops may disrupt hormonal balance in men.

- Chronic alcohol use can affect testosterone and estrogen levels.

Impact on Liver Function

- Alcohol taxes the liver, which also processes fats and proteins from the diet.

- Overconsumption can lead to fatty liver or delayed metabolism of dietary fats.

Personal Decision-Making

Consuming alcohol on a carnivore diet is a matter of personal preference, guided by health goals and cultural context. Key considerations include:

1.   Social and Cultural Factors

Alcohol often facilitates social bonding and celebrations. Abstaining can create feelings of isolation, while moderate consumption can foster a sense of inclusion.

2.   Health and Lifestyle Goals

- Abstinence aligns with optimizing health, metabolism, and mental clarity.

- Moderation allows for enjoyment without significant disruption to diet or health goals.

3.   Mindfulness and Intentionality

- Pay attention to the types and amounts of alcohol consumed.
- Understand that alcohol is a plant-based indulgence and may carry trade-offs beyond its caloric impact.

Practical Tips for Carnivores Who Consume Alcohol

1.   Choose Wisely

- Opt for low-carb options such as dry wines or distilled liquors.
- Avoid beers with gluten and high-carb cocktails.

2.   Moderate Intake

Excess alcohol can lead to metabolic disruption, poor sleep, and impaired recovery.

3.   Hydrate and Replenish

- Alcohol is dehydrating. Drink water before, during, and after consuming alcohol.
- Replenish electrolytes, especially if alcohol disrupts ketosis.

4.   Understand Your Body

- Monitor how alcohol affects your energy, mood, and digestion.
- Consider testing alcohol-free periods to see how abstaining impacts your well-being.

Conclusion: Alcohol as a Conscious Choice

Alcoholic beverages are a unique indulgence that can be enjoyed within the carnivore lifestyle if approached with awareness. While their plant-based origins and metabolic effects may pose challenges, moderation and intentionality allow for occasional participation without significant compromise to health or goals.

> *Whether abstaining or indulging, the key is to remain mindful of the trade-offs and the personal priorities that guide your journey.*

Sugar – Be Careful!

Sugar presents a significant challenge for those who follow a carnivore diet. After a period of avoiding sugar, its effects on the body become much more pronounced, often in startling ways. While many of us previously consumed sugar without immediate or noticeable impact, prolonged abstinence reveals its powerful, often negative influence. This heightened sensitivity is a critical reminder of sugar's potency and potential harm.

The Physical and Psychological Impact of Sugar

1.   Heightened Sensitivity

After sustained avoidance of sugar, indulging in even a small amount— a single cookie or a scoop of ice cream—can result in a pronounced "sugar buzz."

Effects:

- Dizziness and disorientation resembling mild alcohol intoxication.
- Mood swings, from euphoria to irritability as blood sugar spikes and then crashes.
- This sensitivity demonstrates the metabolic stability achieved on a carnivore diet and how easily it can be disrupted.

2.   Blood Sugar Stability

- A meat-centric diet stabilizes blood glucose levels, creating a metabolic environment that is largely unaffected by sugar highs and lows.

- When sugar is introduced, the sudden spike contrasts sharply with this stability, causing discomfort.

Sugar as a Toxin

1.   The Toxic Nature of Sugar

- Sugar's addictive properties and pervasive presence in modern diets make it a subtle but dangerous substance.
- Excessive sugar consumption is linked to metabolic disorders, inflammation, and a range of chronic diseases.

2.   Fructose and Liver Health

Fructose, found in fruits, honey, and high-fructose corn syrup, is metabolized exclusively by the liver.

Risks of Fructose:

- Long-term, repeated exposure to fructose can contribute to non-alcoholic fatty liver disease (NAFLD).
- Overburdening the liver with fructose disrupts its ability to process fats, leading to systemic issues.

Gut Health and Sugar

1.   Unbalanced Gut Microbiome

Sugar feeds harmful bacteria and fungi in the gut, fostering imbalances in the microbiome.

These bacteria can produce toxins that:

- Damage the gut lining, leading to leaky gut syndrome.

- Enter the bloodstream, causing neurological effects such as brain fog, anxiety, or even depression.

2.   Contrast with a Carnivore Diet

A meat-centric diet supports a gut microbiome that thrives on amino acids and fatty acids, reducing inflammation and promoting resilience. Sugar disrupts this balance, often causing discomfort and bloating.

The Exception: Allulose

A Potentially Beneficial Sweetener

- Allulose is a rare sugar with minimal impact on blood glucose and insulin levels.
- Emerging research suggests it may have health benefits, including acting as a GLP-1 agonist, which can help regulate appetite and improve insulin sensitivity.

Caution:

- While promising, the human body has not encountered allulose in significant quantities historically.
- Overuse or reliance on allulose may have unforeseen consequences.

5. Practical Advice for Avoiding Sugar

1.   Reframe Your Perception of Sugar

View sugar not as a harmless treat but as a substance with addictive properties and toxic effects. Consider it a "recreational indulgence" rather than a food.

2.   Be Prepared for Social Situations

Recognize that sugar is ubiquitous in social and celebratory contexts. Politely decline or bring alternatives that align with your lifestyle.

3.   Limit Exposure to Fructose

Avoid sugary fruits, especially high-fructose varieties like apples, grapes, and mangoes. Treat honey and other natural sweeteners with the same caution as processed sugar.

4.   Experiment with Abstinence

Take extended breaks from all forms of sugar to recalibrate your palate and observe its absence on your health and energy.

Conclusion: Sugar and the Carnivore Lifestyle

The longer you stay on a carnivore diet, the clearer sugar's effects become. While it can be challenging to avoid entirely, the benefits of minimizing sugar consumption are profound: stable energy, improved gut health, and reduced risk of chronic disease.

> *Treat sugar with the respect it deserves, understanding its powerful impact on your body and mind. If you choose to indulge, do so sparingly, mindfully, and with full awareness of the trade-offs.*

Meat and Potatoes: Is That Really So Bad?

At first glance, the classic pairing of meat and potatoes seems harmless, even iconic. However, the underlying biochemistry tells a different story. The problem lies in how our bodies process energy.

Our metabolism can derive energy from two primary sources: glucose (from carbohydrates like potatoes) and fat (from foods like meat). **The Randall Cycle**, a metabolic regulatory mechanism, explains why consuming both simultaneously can be problematic.

The Randall Cycle

When glucose and fat are present in high amounts at the same time, the body enters a sort of metabolic traffic jam. **The Randall Cycle** activates to prioritize glucose usage while suppressing fat oxidation. This creates a cascade of effects:

- *Insulin Resistance:* High glucose intake triggers insulin release, which suppresses fat breakdown. Over time, this can contribute to insulin resistance.
- *Fat Storage:* Since fat metabolism is downregulated in the presence of glucose, dietary fats are more likely to be stored as body fat rather than burned for energy.
- *Inflammation:* The metabolic tug-of-war can lead to higher oxidative stress, contributing to systemic inflammation.
- *Energy Crashes:* While glucose provides quick energy, it lacks the sustained, steady supply offered by fat metabolism, leading to fluctuations in energy levels.

From an evolutionary perspective, humans evolved to metabolize fats or carbohydrates efficiently—but not both simultaneously. Historical diets often alternated between periods of higher fat intake and higher carbohydrate intake, rather than combining the two in the same meal.

So, *while meat and potatoes might taste delicious, their biochemical clash can lead to metabolic dysfunction over time*, particularly if consumed frequently. *A better option?* Pairing your protein with healthy fats to stay in the fat-burning zone, or enjoying carbohydrates on rare occasions in isolation when your body is ready to switch to glucose metabolism.

> *This doesn't mean you can never indulge in a nostalgic meal— but understanding the science can help you make more informed decisions about your health.*

THE DILEMMAS
SOCIAL CONSEQUENCES

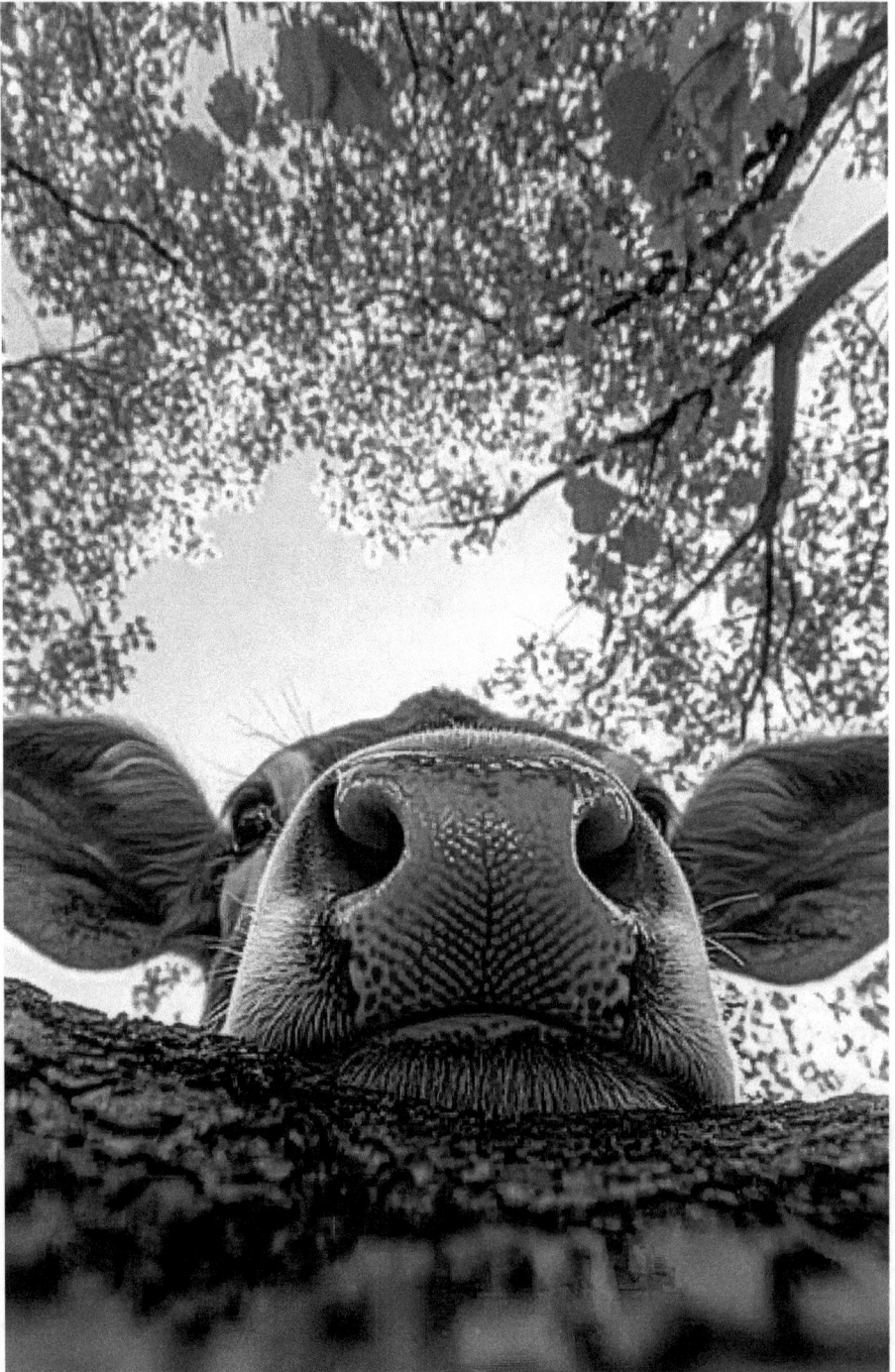

The Sustainability and Ethics of Meat Consumption

The debate over meat consumption is often framed as a binary argument: eating animals is cruel and environmentally harmful, while plant-based diets are ethical and sustainable. But reality is rarely so simple. This section explores the uncomfortable truths and ethical challenges of our food choices, questioning whether the widely accepted narratives about plant agriculture and meat production hold up under scrutiny.

The Ethical Paradox: Is Killing Animals Inherently Cruel?

Humane Practices: Killing animals for food is often labeled as cruel, but the ethical dimension shifts when we consider how livestock is raised and treated. Humane farming practices emphasize providing animals with a life that respects their natural behaviors, access to open spaces, and freedom from unnecessary suffering. Ethical slaughter practices aim to minimize pain and fear, ensuring the process is as quick and humane as possible. For many, eating meat from responsibly raised animals aligns with a moral obligation to treat them with dignity.

Natural Predation: Humans are part of the natural food chain, a reality that often gets overlooked in debates about meat consumption. In nature, predation is an essential force that maintains ecological balance. Carnivorous species rely on other animals for survival, and humans, with their omnivorous physiology, evolved to do the same. From this perspective, eating meat is neither unnatural nor inherently immoral — it reflects our role in the natural world.

Unseen Deaths in Plant Agriculture: Large-scale plant farming isn't as harmless as it seems. Harvesting crops like wheat, corn, and soy involves machinery that inadvertently kills countless small mammals, birds, and insects. Beyond that, destroying natural habitats to make way for fields and applying pesticides leads to further loss of life. These hidden consequences are rarely considered in ethical discussions but are essential to understanding the broader impact of food systems.

Environmental Trade-Offs: Meat vs. Plants

Regenerative Agriculture: Unlike industrial farming, which often damages ecosystems, regenerative agriculture leverages livestock to restore soil health. Grazing animals mimic the natural movement of wild herds, fertilizing the land with their manure and helping sequester carbon in the soil. This approach reduces greenhouse gases and improves biodiversity, offering an alternative to the destructive monocropping practices used for many plant-based foods.

Resource Allocation: Industrial meat production, particularly in CAFOs (Confined Animal Feeding Operations), is resource-intensive. Animals in these systems are fed large amounts of grain and soy, which require extensive land, water, and energy to produce. By contrast, small-scale livestock raised on natural pastures use fewer external resources and provide a sustainable protein source. Redirecting resources away from industrial-scale farming toward regenerative systems can benefit both the environment and food security.

Scale Matters: When considering sustainability, the scale of production is key. Industrial agriculture—whether plant- or animal-based—has significant environmental downsides. However, small-scale, sustainable meat farming can have a lower ecological footprint compared to industrial crop farming. For example, monocropping depletes soil nutrients, requires heavy chemical inputs, and contributes to deforestation, while responsibly raised livestock can complement ecosystems.

Moral Balance: Reconciling Our Role as Meat Eaters

Personal Responsibility: As consumers, we have the power to make choices that align with our values. Supporting farmers who practice ethical animal husbandry and avoiding industrially produced meat are ways to reduce harm. By taking responsibility for the impact of our dietary choices, we can ensure our actions reflect our ethics.

Questioning the 'Plant-Based Savior' Narrative: Plant-based diets are often seen as kinder and more sustainable, but this view ignores the unintended consequences of industrial plant farming. Monocropping destroys ecosystems, reduces biodiversity, and often exploits labor in developing countries. By recognizing these issues, we can move beyond simplistic narratives and embrace a more nuanced understanding of sustainability.

Finding Harmony: Living as a responsible carnivore means balancing personal health with environmental and ethical considerations. While no diet is free from impact, choosing sustainably raised meat and avoiding waste allows us to honor the lives of the animals we consume and the planet we share. By focusing on harmony rather than absolutes, we can find peace in our role as conscious meat eaters.

Conclusion

The sustainability and ethics of meat consumption is a complex dilemma, one that defies easy answers. Carnivores may face criticism for their food choices, but the truth is far more nuanced than slogans or social media soundbites suggest.

By prioritizing humane practices and sustainable systems, we can take responsibility for our impact on the world while aligning with a lifestyle that supports our health and well-being.

If Plants Are Genuinely Toxic, Why Are They So Prevalent in Human Diets?

This topic confronts an uncomfortable but fascinating truth: the dominance of plant-based foods in human diets has historical, economic, and societal underpinnings that go far beyond their actual nutritional value. While plants are abundant and accessible, their widespread consumption reflects compromises and trade-offs made throughout human history rather than an unequivocal endorsement of their superiority for health.

The Historical Context of Plant Consumption

1.   Agriculture and Human Civilization

Agriculture's Rise: Around 10,000 years ago, the advent of agriculture revolutionized human societies, enabling stationary settlements and the growth of civilizations. This shift was driven by the ability to produce large quantities of calorically dense plant foods like grains and tubers.

Trade-Offs: While agriculture allowed for population growth, it also marked a decline in physical health. Archaeological evidence suggests early agriculturalists were shorter, had more dental problems, and suffered from chronic illnesses compared to their hunter-gatherer predecessors.

2.   Scarcity of Animal Foods

Logistical Challenges: Animal foods are more resource-intensive to produce and require larger land areas per calorie compared to plants. As populations grew, reliance on plants became a necessity to feed the masses.

Seasons and Storage: Plants like grains and legumes can be dried and stored for long periods, providing a stable food source, unlike fresh meat, which spoils quickly without modern preservation methods.

Economic and Societal Forces

1.   Affordability and Accessibility

Cost-Effective Calories: Plants are inexpensive to grow and can feed vast populations, making them attractive from an economic standpoint.

Industrialization of Food: Modern agriculture prioritizes mass production, favoring crops like corn, wheat, and soy, which can be grown, processed, and marketed efficiently.

2.   Centralized Control

Population Management: A predominantly plant-based diet can make populations easier to manage. Plants tend to be less nutrient-dense, leading to lower physical vitality, docility, and reduced independent thought—a potentially advantageous outcome for centralized authorities or societal structures reliant on conformity.

The Nutritional Trade-Off

1.   Plant Toxins and Anti-Nutrients

Defense Mechanisms: Plants contain compounds like oxalates, phytates, lectins, and tannins to deter predators (including humans). While these substances can be tolerated in small amounts, chronic consumption may lead to inflammation, nutrient deficiencies, and other health issues.

Bioavailability: Even beneficial nutrients in plants, such as vitamins and minerals, are often less bioavailable than those in animal products due to these same compounds.

2.   Nutritional Gaps

Essential Nutrients: Plants cannot provide certain essential nutrients like vitamin B12, heme iron, and DHA/EPA, all of which are crucial for human health and are found exclusively or primarily in animal foods.

The Psychological and Cultural Aspect

1.   Plant Foods and Ideology

Cultural Identity: Many societies have built their identities around staple crops (e.g., rice in Asia, corn in the Americas). Over time, these foods became ingrained in tradition and daily life.

Virtue Signaling: Modern vegetarian and vegan movements often position plant-based eating as morally superior, further entrenching the idea of plants as the default food.

2.   Dependency on Familiarity

Most people grow up consuming a plant-heavy diet and are culturally conditioned to see it as "normal" and "healthy." Changing this perception requires not just dietary adjustments but also an overhaul of deeply ingrained beliefs.

The Carnivore Perspective

1.   Independent Thinking

A Carnivore diet often fosters a shift in mindset.

As you prioritize animal foods, you may begin to see plant-based diets not just as nutritionally inferior but as reflective of societal conformity and control.

Many Carnivores report increased mental clarity, physical strength, and self-reliance—qualities that align with a more independent, warrior-like disposition.

2.   "Welcome to the Club"

Embracing Carnivore sets you apart, not just physically but also mentally and socially. The lifestyle encourages you to question long-held assumptions about food, health, and society, fostering a greater sense of self-confidence and purpose.

Advice for Carnivores

1.   Choose Quiet Advocacy

- There's no need to proselytize or condemn others for their dietary choices. Set an example through your health, vitality, and calm confidence.
- Understand that most people will not view plants as toxic, and aggressive advocacy may alienate them further.

2.   Focus on Your Path

Concentrate on your own health and well-being. The Carnivore
lifestyle is deeply personal, and the benefits you experience will speak
for themselves.

Conclusion

Plants dominate human diets due to a confluence of historical necessity,
economic practicality, and cultural conditioning. While they have
played a vital role in human survival and societal development, their
nutritional limitations and potential toxicity highlight the trade-offs
involved.

> *As a Carnivore, you can embrace your choice as a return to a
> more ancestral and optimal way of eating, confident in the
> knowledge that you're charting a path that aligns with your
> health and values.*

People Will Tell You That Your Diet Is Unhealthy

This dynamic highlights one of the key themes of The Carnivore's Dilemma: adopting this lifestyle is not just about food—it's about navigating a world that often resists change while staying true to your own health and authenticity.

When you adopt the carnivore lifestyle, you may find yourself confronted by well-meaning but misinformed critiques from people who are themselves struggling with their health. Friends, family members, colleagues, and even strangers might challenge your choices, citing concerns about cholesterol, heart disease, or the supposed dangers of eating "too much meat."

What makes these interactions fascinating is the disconnect between their stated concerns and their personal realities. Often, these critics:

- Are dealing with chronic health conditions, such as obesity, diabetes, or hypertension.
- Rely on multiple medications to manage their symptoms rather than addressing root causes.
- Struggle with energy, mobility, or endurance compared to your increased vitality on a meat-based diet.

This irony can be perplexing, but it also reveals how deeply ingrained conventional dietary narratives are. Many people unconsciously defend these narratives because they represent a sense of stability and trust in institutional advice, even when their own experiences may suggest otherwise.

Why Does This Happen?

- *Cognitive Dissonance:* Seeing someone thrive on a diet that contradicts mainstream advice can create internal conflict. To resolve this discomfort, people may try to dismiss or discredit the alternative perspective.

- *Cultural Conditioning:* For decades, we've been told that balanced diets must include whole grains, fruits, and vegetables while limiting red meat. Questioning these guidelines can feel like challenging an almost religious belief system.

- *Projection of Fear:* People often project their fears or misunderstandings onto others. Warnings about cholesterol or longevity are frequently rooted in outdated or oversimplified information.

How to Respond

- *Lead by Example:* Your improved health, energy, and strength are powerful rebuttals to criticism. Over time, your success can spark curiosity and open the door for meaningful conversations.

- *Stay Informed:* Equip yourself with knowledge about the science behind the carnivore diet. This allows you to confidently address common misconceptions without becoming confrontational.

- *Choose Your Battles:* Not every critique requires a response. Assess whether the person is genuinely curious or simply defending their beliefs, and engage accordingly.

- *Empathize:* Understand that their comments often come from a place of concern or misunderstanding, not malice. A compassionate approach can defuse tension and create opportunities for dialogue.

Reframing the Criticism

Instead of viewing these interactions as discouraging, consider them opportunities to reflect on your own transformation. The fact that people feel compelled to comment on your lifestyle is a testament to the visible impact it's having. Your journey can challenge others to reevaluate their assumptions, even if they don't openly admit it.

Be Careful with Your Assertiveness

Adopting a carnivore diet often leads to profound changes in the body's biochemistry, with cascading effects on physical health, energy levels, mental clarity, and even personality traits. Many who embrace this lifestyle report shifts that extend beyond the physiological into the realm of self-perception, behavior, and interpersonal dynamics. One of the most intriguing and nuanced aspects of this transformation is the tendency toward increased assertiveness—an unintended yet powerful consequence of better health and hormonal balance.

The Biochemical Basis of Assertiveness

1.   Improved Blood Chemistry

The shift to a meat-centric diet optimizes lipid transport, enhancing the body's ability to deliver energy at a cellular level. The mitochondria, the powerhouses of the cells, transition from a glucose-dominant metabolism to producing ATP via the electron transport chain, a far more efficient process. This energy surplus often translates into heightened vitality, focus, and decisiveness.

2.   Hormonal Rebalancing

A meat-first diet provides the body with ample cholesterol, a vital substrate for producing hormones such as testosterone, estrogen, and cortisol. For many, this leads to a restoration of hormonal balance, which can manifest in greater confidence, a stronger sense of purpose, and, in men particularly, an emergence of warrior-like traits and mindsets.

3.   Sharper Mental Clarity

The absence of plant-based irritants and a reliance on nutrient-dense foods can alleviate brain fog, improve emotional stability, and foster a sense of mental sharpness that amplifies one's ability to articulate thoughts and act decisively.

The Assertiveness Dilemma

While these biochemical and hormonal benefits are undoubtedly positive, they can lead to unintended consequences in social and interpersonal settings. For many, the newfound energy and confidence might translate into behaviors that, while natural, could be perceived as overly assertive, domineering, or even abrasive. This is particularly relevant in a modern world that often prizes tact, diplomacy, and emotional subtlety over directness and strength.

1.   Unintentional Domineering

Without proper awareness, the natural assertiveness fostered by this lifestyle might come across as overbearing, especially to those accustomed to a more subdued or conventional demeanor.

2.   Shifting Social Dynamics

Others may interpret this change as arrogance or aggression, leading to misunderstandings or strained relationships, especially in settings where assertive behavior is not the norm.

The Opportunity to Manage and Refine Assertiveness

The heightened energy, confidence, and clarity that accompany the carnivore diet offer an opportunity for personal growth—if managed wisely. These changes invite practitioners to cultivate self-awareness and develop the skills to channel their newfound strength constructively.

1.   Practicing Mindful Communication

Recognizing the impact of words and tone is crucial. Assertiveness should be paired with empathy and active listening to ensure that interactions are collaborative rather than confrontational.

2.   Balancing Strength with Respect

Embodying the warrior mindset doesn't necessitate conflict. Instead, it involves leading with strength while remaining respectful and considerate of others' perspectives.

3.   Harnessing Confidence for Positive Influence

Increased self-assurance can be a powerful tool for inspiring and motivating others. By framing assertiveness as a means of empowerment rather than dominance, carnivores can use their energy to build stronger relationships and foster mutual respect.

4.   Learning Emotional Intelligence

Greater assertiveness also comes with the responsibility to understand the emotions and boundaries of those around you. Developing emotional intelligence helps temper directness with sensitivity, ensuring interactions remain positive and productive.

A Path of Self-Discovery

The emergence of assertiveness is not a flaw but a reflection of deeper alignment with one's natural state of health and vitality. By learning to channel this energy constructively, carnivores can embrace their newfound capacities as tools for growth and leadership. In doing so, they navigate the delicate balance between authenticity and social harmony, transforming assertiveness from a potential liability into a profound strength.

A Loss of Interest in Romantic Partners Who Are Plant-Eaters

Dietary choices often reflect deeper values, beliefs, and lifestyles. For those transformed by a carnivore diet, these choices can create a divide between themselves and romantic partners who adhere to plant-based eating. While this is a sensitive and personal topic, it highlights the profound impact of dietary alignment—or misalignment—on relationships, particularly when food represents more than mere sustenance.

Evolving Perceptions of Plant-Based Eating

1.   Viewing Plant-Eaters as Weak or Unhealthy

As carnivores experience significant health transformations, including greater energy, mental clarity, and physical resilience, they may perceive plant-based diets as inherently limiting or harmful. Witnessing the struggles of plant-eaters—such as frequent illness, reliance on supplements, or mood instability—can make their dietary choices seem unappealing or misguided.

2.   A Clash of Values

Carnivores often embrace their diet as a statement of strength, self-reliance, and authenticity. By contrast, they may interpret plant-based eating as emblematic of societal conformity, health misinformation, or a rejection of ancestral wisdom. These conflicting perspectives can create tension, especially when diet becomes a core aspect of personal identity.

The Disconnection of Shared Meals

1.   Food as a Source of Togetherness

Food is a cornerstone of human connection, often serving as a ritual that fosters intimacy and mutual understanding. For carnivores, meals centered on plant-based foods may feel like a disconnect rather than a point of togetherness. The inability to share a dietary worldview during something as fundamental as eating can diminish the shared experience of a relationship.

2.   Daily Frictions

Beyond shared meals, dietary incompatibility can spill into other aspects of life. Grocery shopping, meal preparation, dining out, and even discussing food choices can become sources of friction rather than joy.

The Challenge of Respecting Differences

1.   Sensitivity to Individual Choices

While a carnivore may view plant-based eating as flawed, respecting a partner's autonomy and beliefs is essential for maintaining emotional intimacy. This can be especially challenging when dietary choices feel at odds with one's own values or worldview.

2.   Balancing Acceptance and Authenticity

Navigating these differences often requires striking a delicate balance between honoring a partner's dietary decisions and staying true to one's own identity. Carnivores may struggle with how much compromise is acceptable without feeling they are betraying their own principles.

The Path Forward

1.   Fostering Understanding

While dietary differences can be challenging, open communication and mutual curiosity can bridge gaps. Sharing the reasons behind one's dietary choices without judgment and listening to a partner's perspective can foster greater empathy and respect.

2.   Seeking Alignment

For some carnivores, compatibility in diet and lifestyle becomes non-negotiable. In such cases, seeking a partner who shares similar views on health, food, and values may provide a stronger foundation for connection and shared purpose.

A Sensitive Yet Transformative Aspect

The loss of interest in romantic partners who are plant-eaters reflects the profound ways a carnivore lifestyle reshapes identity, values, and preferences. While it can create tension or even distance in relationships, it also offers an opportunity for deeper self-discovery and clarity about what one seeks in a partnership.

Ultimately, this aspect of the carnivore journey challenges individuals to navigate complex emotional and relational terrain, balancing personal authenticity with respect for others' choices. For those who find alignment in both diet and values, the rewards can be a deeper sense of connection, understanding, and shared purpose.

Going to Social Outings Where Food Is Central

For carnivores, social outings centered on food may initially seem daunting but tend to become manageable with preparation and the right mindset. These gatherings often present challenges in terms of available options, dietary understanding, and interpersonal dynamics. However, with thoughtful strategies and a calm approach, they can become an opportunity to enjoy connection without conflict.

Be Prepared and Self-Sufficient

1.   Bring Your Own Food

Preparation is key. Carrying portable, carnivore-friendly snacks such as meat sticks, jerky, or pre-cooked meats ensures that you have something to enjoy, even if the offerings are unsuitable. This simple act removes stress and allows you to focus on socializing rather than navigating limited food choices.

2.   Assess the Menu in Advance

For events at restaurants or catered gatherings, reviewing the menu beforehand can be helpful. Many establishments are willing to make modifications, such as serving meat without sauces or side dishes. A polite request ensures you can eat comfortably while minimizing attention to your dietary choices.

Navigating Questions and Comments

1.   Addressing Curiosity

Social outings may spark questions or comments from those unfamiliar with the carnivore lifestyle. People often express curiosity or skepticism, ranging from genuine interest to awkward or even judgmental remarks.

- A calm, brief response—such as "I've found this way of eating works best for me"—often suffices.
- Avoid over-explaining or debating, as this can unintentionally put others on the defensive, especially plant-eaters.

2.   Setting a Positive Example

Your demeanor can speak volumes. Demonstrating confidence, ease, and good-natured acceptance of your dietary choices sets a positive tone. It shows that you can enjoy the event without making food the focal point of potential discord.

Respecting the Efforts of Others

1.   Accommodations by Hosts

Friends, family, or hosts may try to accommodate your diet, often with the best intentions. However, their understanding may be limited, and their offerings may not align with your preferences.

- Graciously acknowledge their effort, even if you choose not to partake.
- A polite "Thank you, but I'll stick with what I brought" can avoid awkwardness while maintaining your boundaries.

2. Avoiding Dietary Advocacy

While you may be enthusiastic about the benefits of carnivory, social outings are rarely the place for advocacy. Attempts to convince others, however well-meaning, may come across as critical or alienating. Focusing on shared enjoyment rather than dietary differences helps maintain harmony.

Shifting Focus Away from Food

1.   Emphasizing Connection

Food may be central to the gathering, but it doesn't have to dominate your experience. Redirect your attention to the conversations, activities, or company present. This approach shifts the focus from dietary constraints to meaningful engagement with others.

2.   Remaining Flexible

Unexpected circumstances are bound to arise, but maintaining a flexible and unflustered attitude allows you to adapt. For instance, you might eat a meal before the event and focus on beverages or light snacks during the outing.

The Bigger Picture

1.   Building Social Confidence

As you navigate more social outings, you may find that the challenges become less significant. Each experience builds confidence and equips you with tools to handle future situations with greater ease.

2.   Setting an Example of Ease and Health

By participating fully in social events without making your diet a source of contention, you embody the benefits of the carnivore lifestyle. Your good mood, vitality, and calm acceptance can leave a lasting impression far more powerful than words.

Navigating with Grace and Poise

Social outings where food is central don't have to be stressful or alienating. With preparation, a positive attitude, and respect for others' perspectives, these events can become enjoyable occasions for connection. By focusing on relationships and shared experiences rather than dietary differences, you demonstrate the adaptability and confidence that are hallmarks of a thriving carnivore lifestyle.

Do You Try to Convince Others to Take on Carnivore?

The dilemma of whether or not to advocate for the Carnivore lifestyle is a challenging one. On one hand, the profound benefits you've experienced may inspire a genuine desire to help others improve their health and well-being. On the other hand, such conversations can often be met with resistance, misunderstanding, or outright hostility, especially when deeply ingrained beliefs or personal values are challenged.

The Desire to Share

1.   Personal Transformation

- When Carnivore leads to increased vitality, mental clarity, and physical health, it's natural to want to share this "secret" with others.
- Particularly with loved ones, there is often an urge to help them find solutions to health challenges you believe Carnivore could address.

2.   The Problem of Enthusiasm

- Enthusiasm, while well-meaning, can be perceived as overbearing or judgmental.
- Attempts to explain or advocate for Carnivore may inadvertently come across as dismissive of other lifestyles, particularly plant-based or mixed diets.

Common Reactions from Others

1.   Repulsion

- Many people find the idea of a meat-exclusive diet repugnant, whether for ethical, environmental, or health reasons.
- Visuals of large quantities of meat or the rejection of fruits and vegetables can trigger strong reactions.

2.   Skepticism

- Many are conditioned to believe that plant-based diets are the healthiest and that red meat, in particular, is harmful.
- Without a willingness to explore evidence or question mainstream dietary guidelines, they may dismiss Carnivore as unsafe or pseudoscientific.

3.   Offense

- Advocacy for Carnivore often entails criticism of plant-based diets, even if unintentional.
- Statements about the dangers of oxalates, anti-nutrients, or fructose can feel like personal attacks on someone who believes they are making healthy choices.

Why Advocating for Carnivore Can Be Problematic

1.   Conflict of Worldviews

- Diets are deeply tied to identity, culture, and ethical values.
- Suggesting that someone's dietary approach is flawed can feel like questioning their core beliefs.

2.   Lack of a Shared Starting Point

Without shared knowledge of nutrition, physiology, or the Carnivore rationale, it's easy for discussions to devolve into emotional arguments.

3.   Social Dynamics

Bringing up dietary differences can create tension in relationships, especially when others feel judged or pressured.

Strategies for Navigating the Dilemma

1.   Lead by Example

• Be a Living Testament
• The best way to inspire curiosity and interest is to simply live the lifestyle and embody its benefits.
• When others see your energy, health, and satisfaction, they may naturally ask questions out of curiosity rather than defensiveness.

2.   Gauge Interest

• Speak Only When Asked
• Share your experience only when someone expresses genuine interest or curiosity.
• Avoid unsolicited advice or explanations that may seem preachy.

3.   Use Neutral Language

• Avoid Confrontation
• Frame Carnivore as a personal choice rather than a superior one.
• Example: "This works really well for me" instead of "This is the best way to eat."

4.   Focus on Common Ground

Health and Well-Being

- Emphasize shared goals like improving health, energy, or weight management.
- Discuss concepts that may resonate universally, such as reducing processed foods.

5.   Be Prepared for Criticism

- Stay Calm
- Expect skepticism or even ridicule, and don't take it personally.
- Understand that resistance often comes from misinformation or emotional ties to other diets.

When Advocacy May Be Necessary

There are times when discussing Carnivore might be appropriate or even important:

- With Loved Ones Facing Health Challenges: If someone close to you is struggling with health issues that Carnivore might alleviate, gentle advocacy could be life-changing.
- In Close Relationships: Romantic partners or household members may need to understand your lifestyle to foster harmony.

In these cases, approach the conversation with empathy and respect. Share information gradually, allowing the other person to explore at their own pace.

Conclusion: Choose Your Battles

Advocating for Carnivore is a double-edged sword. While the desire to share its benefits is natural, the potential for conflict is high. Focus on leading by example and letting your results speak for themselves.

> *Engage others only when they show genuine interest, and remember that every person's journey is their own. Respect for autonomy and diversity in dietary choices is key to maintaining positive relationships while living true to your values.*

On Vegetarians: Navigating Differences with Grace

Vegetarians can present a unique challenge for those living a Carnivore lifestyle. Often passionate about their choices, they may express their views in ways that feel confrontational, self-righteous, or dismissive. Their strong beliefs about the ethical, environmental, or health superiority of a plant-based diet can lead to tense interactions, especially if they perceive Carnivore as antithetical to their values. However, how we respond to these situations matters greatly—not just for preserving relationships but also for demonstrating the confidence and peace that can come from fully embracing Carnivore.

Avoiding the Trap of Hostility

1.   Don't Mirror Negative Behavior

- If a vegetarian adopts a pedantic or hostile tone, resist the urge to match it.
- Stay calm, respectful, and self-assured. Reacting emotionally diminishes your credibility and can escalate tensions unnecessarily.

2.   Reject Self-Righteousness

- Avoid falling into the same trap of moral superiority.
- While you may strongly believe in the benefits of Carnivore, remember that dietary choices are deeply personal and often tied to one's values, upbringing, or identity.

The Power of Quiet Confidence

1.   Let Your Results Speak

- Be a "quiet champion." Allow the physical, mental, and emotional benefits you've experienced to be your primary advocacy.
- People are more likely to be curious about your lifestyle when they see its positive impact on you rather than hear it from you unsolicited.

2.   No Need for Proselytizing

- Unlike those who may feel the need to reconvince themselves of their choices through constant advocacy, a truly content Carnivore has no such compulsion.
- Confidence in your path diminishes the need for external validation.

Strategies for Peaceful Coexistence

1.   Embrace Empathy

- Understand that vegetarians are often motivated by deeply held beliefs—whether ethical, environmental, or health-related.
- Their hostility may stem from feeling their values are being challenged, not necessarily from personal animosity.

2.   Find Common Ground

- Highlight shared goals like health, sustainability, or animal welfare (e.g., humane sourcing).
- Avoid framing the conversation as "us vs. them." Instead, focus on how your approach works for you without devaluing theirs.

3.   Deflect and Redirect

If confronted, stay non-confrontational:

Example: "I've found what works best for me, and I respect that you've done the same."

This approach closes the door to arguments while affirming mutual respect.

When to Engage and When to Walk Away

1.   Engage Sparingly

- Only dive deeper into discussions if the other party is open-minded and genuinely curious.
- Avoid debates with individuals who are firmly entrenched in their views—it's unlikely to be productive.

2.   Know When to Exit

If the conversation turns hostile or circular, politely disengage: "I think we're coming at this from very different perspectives, and that's okay."

Why You Shouldn't Be Like "Them"

1.   Live Your Values Without Preaching

- Unlike a proselytizing vegetarian, who may need constant affirmation of their choices, a secure Carnivore radiates assurance without needing to impose their beliefs.
- Your lifestyle is your statement—it doesn't require a podium or a debate.

2.   Show What True Confidence Looks Like

By being calm, kind, and respectful, you showcase the strength and clarity that comes from a fulfilled, intentional life.

Conclusion: Coexisting with Vegetarians

The Carnivore-vegetarian divide doesn't have to be fraught with conflict. By adopting a mindset of quiet confidence, leading by example, and avoiding unnecessary debates, you can coexist peacefully with vegetarians—even those who may be hostile or critical.

> *Remember, the goal isn't to convert others but to live authentically, demonstrating the benefits of your lifestyle through your own contentment and results.*

People Will Tell You That You Are Too Thin

One of the more common criticisms you may face on the Carnivore diet is that you are "too thin." This remark often stems from conventional ideas about body composition, appearance, and even health. For those who embrace Carnivore, where weight naturally normalizes to a leaner state, these comments can be surprising or even frustrating. Addressing this dilemma requires both self-awareness and thoughtful communication.

Why This Happens

1.   Modern Standards of "Healthy"

- Many people equate health with a soft, fuller body, influenced by societal norms shaped by a carb-centric diet. A lean, muscular, or slender frame may seem "too thin" by comparison.
- Chronic inflammation, water retention, and higher fat stores are so normalized that a healthy, lean body can appear unfamiliar or concerning.

2.   Projection of Their Own Insecurities

Comments about your weight often reflect others' insecurities or misunderstandings rather than a genuine assessment of your health.

3.   Carnivore's Impact on Body Composition

Carnivore naturally shifts the body toward optimal fat-to-muscle ratios. This often results in a leaner, healthier frame that may not align with the broader population's perception of "normal."

How to Respond

1.   Stay Calm and Confident

- Remind yourself that these comments are usually well-meaning but uninformed.
- Acknowledge their concern without internalizing it: "I appreciate your concern, but I feel great and am confident in my health."

2.   Provide Simple Explanations (if Desired)

- You don't owe anyone a detailed justification, but sometimes a brief response can clarify misconceptions:
- "This is my natural weight on a diet that works for me. I feel healthy, strong, and energetic."
- "A meat-based diet has helped me reach a body composition that feels right for me."

3.   Avoid Arguments

Resist the urge to dive into debates or defend your choices. Often, this leads to misunderstandings or heightened tensions.

Focus on Your Own Perception

1.   Trust Your Body

- Weight loss or a leaner appearance on Carnivore is typically a reflection of reduced inflammation, improved metabolism, and hormonal balance.
- If you feel healthy, energetic, and strong, your body is likely thriving — even if it doesn't match societal norms.

2.   Health Over Appearance

Remember that true health is not determined by external opinions but by how you feel and function. Lab work, physical performance, and overall well-being are better indicators of health than the number on the scale or others' perceptions.

Navigating Social Situations

1.   When Family and Friends Comment

Close relationships may come with more persistent or emotionally charged remarks. A reassuring response might be: "I've found something that works for me and helps me feel my best. My weight is just a natural outcome of this lifestyle."

2.   Public or Casual Remarks

For less personal interactions, you can simply deflect: "This is what works for me."

3.   Lead by Example

Over time, your consistent energy, mood, and vitality will often speak louder than words.

A Broader Perspective

1.   Challenging Conventional Beliefs

- The notion that lean equals unhealthy is deeply ingrained but often misguided. Many populations with lower body fat percentages are among the healthiest and longest-lived.

- By embracing your Carnivore lifestyle, you challenge norms and redefine what health can look like.

2.   Redefining "Too Thin"

Weight that results from eating nutrient-dense, animal-based foods and avoiding processed carbohydrates is likely closer to your biological ideal than the societal "average."

When to Seek Reassurance

Listen to Your Body: If you're unsure whether your weight loss is healthy, consult a knowledgeable doctor or track markers like energy levels, strength, and lab results.

Stay Open to Adjustments: If you genuinely feel you've lost too much weight, increasing fat intake, adding more calories, or diversifying your animal-based foods may help.

Conclusion

When people tell you that you're "too thin," recognize it as an opportunity to educate or simply dismiss it with quiet confidence. As long as you feel strong, healthy, and vibrant, your weight is likely a reflection of the incredible benefits of Carnivore.

> *Remember, your journey is about optimizing your health and well-being—not meeting others' expectations.*

THE DILEMMAS
BEING CARNIVORE

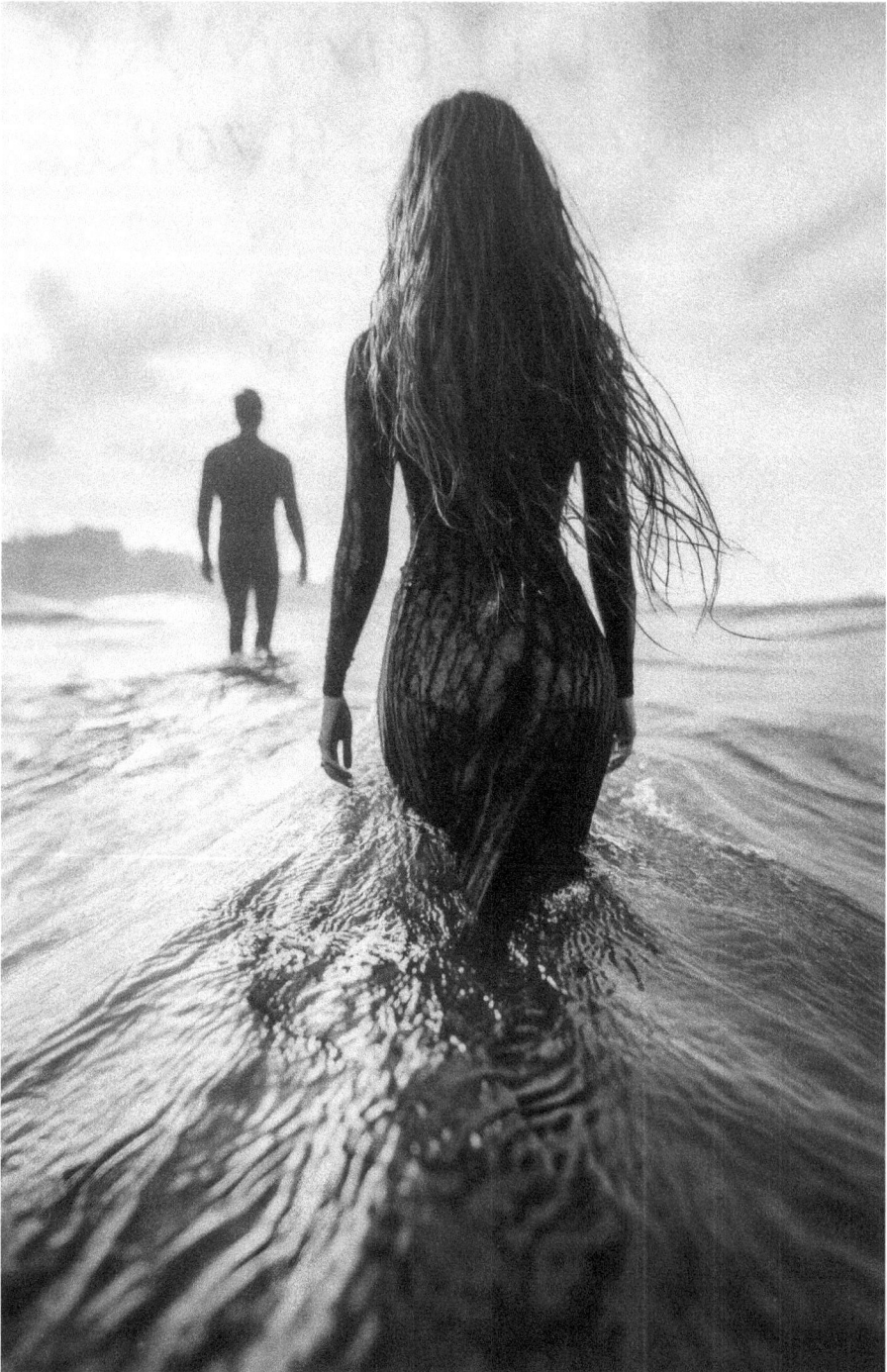

The Personal Journey of Being Carnivore

Being Carnivore is not a one-size-fits-all blueprint but a deeply personal journey of discovery, adaptation, and refinement. Each individual's experience is unique, shaped by physiology, goals, circumstances, and values.

Being Carnivore is as much about the process of discovery as it is about the destination. By taking the time to understand your body, adapt to challenges, and craft a lifestyle that resonates with your personal values and goals, you can unlock the full potential of this transformative path.

Here's what to consider as you navigate this transformative lifestyle...

Discovering What Works Best for You

Listening to Your Body: Every person's physiology is different. What works well for one Carnivore may not work as effectively for another. For instance, some thrive on a strict beef-and-water diet, while others incorporate seafood, eggs, or occasional dairy. The key is to pay attention to how your body responds — energy levels, digestion, mental clarity, and overall well-being — and adjust your approach accordingly.

Trial and Adjustment: The Carnivore lifestyle requires experimentation. It's a process of learning what foods you tolerate well, what ratios of fat to protein suit your energy needs, and how to balance enjoyment with sustainability. There's no rush; discovering your unique path takes time.

Adapting Over Time

Physiological Adaptation: Transitioning to Carnivore involves a period of physical adjustment as your body adapts to burning fat for fuel instead of carbohydrates. This process, often called becoming "fat-adapted," may involve temporary discomforts such as fatigue or cravings. These challenges are normal and typically resolve as your metabolism shifts. Patience is key.

Psychological Growth: Moving to a Carnivore lifestyle often means unlearning years of dietary conditioning. Psychological adaptation involves embracing new habits, questioning ingrained beliefs about food, and cultivating a sense of confidence in your choices. This can be both empowering and liberating.

Social Adaptation: Navigating social settings as a Carnivore can be challenging. Family dinners, restaurant outings, and holidays often center around plant-heavy dishes or processed foods. Over time, you'll develop strategies to handle these situations gracefully—whether that means bringing your own food, politely declining certain dishes, or finding creative ways to enjoy social occasions without compromising your choices.

Deciding How to Live as a Carnivore

Degrees of Restriction: The beauty of the Carnivore lifestyle lies in its flexibility. Some individuals find joy and simplicity in strict adherence, consuming only animal-based foods. Others allow occasional indulgences—like a piece of dark chocolate or a glass of wine—while maintaining the core principles of the diet. There's no "right" way to do Carnivore; the balance is yours to define.

Balancing Enjoyment and Longevity: Life is about more than dietary perfection. While optimal health and vitality are crucial, so is savoring the moments that bring happiness. For some, this might mean a rare indulgence in a favorite non-Carnivore dish or finding ways to incorporate cherished traditions into the lifestyle. The ultimate goal is a life that is both enjoyable and sustainable.

Embracing the Long View

Sustainability of Choice: Choosing the Carnivore lifestyle is not about perfection but about progress. Over time, you'll find a rhythm that feels natural and sustainable for you. This journey isn't a sprint—it's a lifelong commitment to health, self-discovery, and living in alignment with your values.

Evolving as You Go: Your Carnivore path may change as your body, circumstances, and goals evolve. It's okay to adjust your approach, experiment with new foods, or reevaluate your choices over time. The journey is dynamic, not static.

Finding Joy in the Journey

Celebrating Wins: Whether it's improved energy, better mental clarity, or weight loss, take time to celebrate the milestones you achieve along the way. These moments reinforce your commitment and highlight the benefits of your efforts.

Connection and Support: Joining the Carnivore community—whether online or in person—can provide invaluable support, inspiration, and camaraderie. Sharing your experiences and learning from others can make the journey even more rewarding.

Leadership and Partnership in the Carnivore Journey

Becoming the Leader of Your Own Health

The Carnivore lifestyle requires a level of self-leadership that goes beyond conventional dietary practices. In a world where mainstream narratives often contradict the principles of a meat-first diet, embracing Carnivore means taking responsibility for your own health and well-being. Being a leader for yourself involves:

Educating Yourself: It's essential to deepen your knowledge about metabolism, nutrition, and the science behind the Carnivore approach. This empowers you to see through misinformation and advocate for your health with confidence.

Critical Thinking: Recognize that mainstream dietary guidelines are often shaped by political, economic, and industrial influences. By understanding the deeper truths behind health and nutrition, you can make informed decisions that align with your goals.

Conducting N=1 Experiments: Leadership involves curiosity and experimentation. By observing how your body responds to specific foods, exceptions, or transgressions, you can fine-tune your approach. These self-directed experiments help you identify what works best and what hinders your progress.

> *As a self-leader, you are not just following a diet—you are actively crafting a lifestyle tailored to your unique needs, values, and aspirations.*

The Power of Partnership

While self-leadership is vital, the Carnivore journey becomes richer and more sustainable when shared with a partner or friend. The path can be isolating in a world that often questions or misunderstands this lifestyle. A trusted companion offers support, camaraderie, and a shared sense of purpose.

Partnership provides:

Mutual Encouragement: Having someone to share successes and setbacks can help maintain motivation, especially during moments of doubt or difficulty.

Shared Knowledge: Discussing evolving understandings, discoveries, and resources enhances both partners' learning and growth.

Collaborative Experimentation: Conducting experiments together— trying new foods, exploring fasting protocols, or testing supplements— can lead to deeper insights and a stronger bond.

Social Ease: Navigating social situations is easier when you're not alone. A partner can help normalize your choices in shared settings and provide a sense of solidarity.

> *Partnership doesn't have to be limited to a romantic partner or close friend. Connecting with a larger Carnivore community— whether online or in person—can create a network of support and inspiration that helps sustain you through the challenges.*

Leadership and Partnership in Harmony

Ultimately, being Carnivore is about striking a balance between independence and connection. Self-leadership allows you to take charge of your health, while partnership ensures you have the support and collaboration needed to thrive. Together, these aspects create a strong foundation for success in navigating the challenges of a meat-first lifestyle.

> *Whether you lead yourself with unwavering determination or walk the path hand-in-hand with others, this journey is one of empowerment, discovery, and growth.*

Attitudes About Hygiene May Change, Radically

One of the more unexpected shifts experienced by those who adopt a carnivore diet is a transformation in attitudes toward personal hygiene. This change stems largely from the profound effects the diet has on body chemistry and the microbiome. Many hygiene practices considered essential in modern society—like frequent tooth brushing, the use of deodorants, or meticulous skin care routines—may become less relevant or even counterproductive as the body adapts to this nutrient-dense, low-toxin way of eating.

The Carnivore Impact on Body Chemistry and Biome

1.   Improved Oral Health

A meat-first diet eliminates the primary culprits behind tooth decay and gum disease: sugars and plant-based carbohydrates. These foods feed harmful bacteria in the mouth, leading to plaque buildup, cavities, and other dental issues. With their removal, many carnivores report cleaner teeth, reduced plaque, and fresher breath even without frequent brushing or the use of toothpaste.

2.   Changes in Body Odor

The absence of plant-based compounds, particularly those high in sulfur or oxalates, results in a noticeable change in body odor. Carnivores often find that they sweat less or that their sweat has a more neutral scent, reducing the need for deodorants or frequent showers.

3.   Healthier Skin

By eliminating inflammatory foods, the carnivore diet may alleviate
conditions like acne, eczema, or dryness. The skin often becomes less
reactive and more balanced, reducing the need for skincare products or
elaborate cleansing routines.

4.   A Balanced Microbiome

Without the fiber and plant antinutrients that disrupt gut bacteria, the
microbiome may stabilize. This balance affects the entire body,
including skin and oral health, contributing to a cleaner, healthier
appearance with less intervention.

Reevaluating Hygiene Norms

For many, this shift challenges deeply ingrained societal norms about
cleanliness. Modern hygiene practices often revolve around managing
the side effects of a high-carb, plant-heavy diet—frequent tooth
brushing to combat sugar-related decay, deodorants to mask odors
caused by metabolic waste, or skincare to address inflammation from
dietary irritants. When the underlying causes of these issues are
addressed, the "need" for such practices diminishes.

Navigating the Change

1.   Adapting Hygiene Routines

Carnivores may find themselves questioning the necessity of traditional
hygiene routines. For example, tooth brushing might shift from a twice-
daily ritual with toothpaste to a simpler cleaning routine. Similarly,
fewer showers or a reduction in skincare products may suffice to
maintain a fresh and healthy appearance.

2.   Overcoming Social Expectations

Shifting hygiene habits may draw curiosity or concern from others. Explaining the rationale behind these changes—or simply being confident in one's choices—can help navigate social interactions gracefully.

3.   Understanding the Science

Educating oneself about the biochemistry behind these changes can foster confidence and provide evidence-based responses to skepticism or questions.

The Broader Implications

This radical shift in hygiene highlights a deeper transformation: the carnivore lifestyle not only changes what we consume but also how we engage with the world around us. By addressing the root causes of many modern hygiene concerns, it invites a simpler, more natural approach to self-care—one that reflects the body's inherent ability to maintain balance and health when properly nourished.

> *For many, this shift is liberating, offering freedom from reliance on products and routines that once felt obligatory. It exemplifies how profoundly the carnivore diet can reshape perceptions of the body, health, and what it means to be truly clean.*

A Feeling of Revoltingness at Plants-as-Food

One of the more striking evolutions many carnivores experience is a growing sense of aversion toward plant-based foods. This shift often occurs as the body and mind adapt to a meat-centric diet, where cravings for plants diminish and, in some cases, transform into outright repugnance. This phenomenon is neither a matter of psychological rejection nor an arbitrary preference—it often reflects a deeper physiological response.

The Shift in Desire

1.   Diminished Cravings

As the body normalizes to nutrient-dense animal-based foods, the allure of plants fades. Foods that were once staples, such as vegetables, grains, or sugary fruits, may no longer seem desirable. For many carnivores, this shift feels effortless: the body's innate signals align with its nutritional needs, eliminating the need for restraint or discipline.

2.   Association with Discomfort

For those who occasionally reintroduce plant-based foods, the results are often telling. Many report digestive disturbances, brain fog, inflammation, or a general sense of unwellness following consumption. Over time, this negative reinforcement creates a natural tendency to avoid plants altogether.

A Physiological Basis

1.   The Body's Response

The human digestive system and metabolic processes adjust
significantly on a carnivore diet. Without plant antinutrients—like
lectins, oxalates, and phytates—gut health improves, inflammation
decreases, and overall well-being increases. Reintroducing these
compounds can provoke noticeable discomfort, reinforcing the aversion
to plants.

2.   Taste and Texture Changes

As taste buds recalibrate, the flavors and textures of plant-based foods
may become less appealing. Bitter or fibrous plants, in particular, might
trigger a visceral sense of rejection as the body instinctively associates
them with potential harm or poor nutritional value.

The Role of Adaptation

1.   Beyond Addiction

Many modern diets foster an addiction-like relationship with plant-
based foods, particularly those high in sugar, caffeine, or processed
additives. Breaking free from this dependency on a carnivore diet
allows the body to reset, revealing its true preferences and needs.

2.   An Evolutionary Perspective

From an evolutionary standpoint, plants often served as survival foods
rather than primary sources of nutrition. This historical relationship
may help explain why, once the body thrives on animal-based nutrition,
it no longer seeks out or tolerates plants.

Navigating the Aversion

1.   Social Implications

Expressing a newfound distaste for plants can be challenging in social settings, where vegetables or plant-based dishes are often central to meals. Carnivores may need to find tactful ways to navigate these scenarios without offending hosts or drawing undue attention.

2.   Personal Growth

Accepting and embracing this aversion can be an empowering part of the carnivore journey. It signifies a deeper connection to the body's signals and a rejection of societal norms that promote plants as essential or superior foods.

A Deeper Transformation

The aversion to plants as food marks a profound physiological and psychological shift. It reflects not just a change in dietary preference but a deeper alignment with what nourishes and sustains the body. For many, this newfound clarity provides a sense of liberation—free from cravings, guilt, or the pervasive dietary dogmas of modern society.

> *Rather than feeling restricted, carnivores often describe this aversion as a natural progression in their journey toward health and well-being. It serves as a reminder that the body, when properly nourished, instinctively knows what it needs and what to avoid.*

How Restrictive Should I Be?

The carnivore diet, like any dietary choice, is highly personal. While it emphasizes animal-based foods, the level of restriction within that framework should be determined by individual needs, health goals, and personal preferences. The beauty of this lifestyle lies in its adaptability, allowing each person to tailor their approach for optimal health and satisfaction.

Carnivore as a Personal Journey

1.   Finding What Works Best for You

There's no universal blueprint for carnivore eating. Some individuals thrive on a strictly meat-and-water regimen, while others incorporate dairy, eggs, or even occasional plant-derived foods. The key is to experiment and discover what makes you feel your best.

2.   Listening to Your Body

Over time, your body will guide your choices. Many carnivores find that as they commit to this lifestyle, their cravings for plant-based foods diminish naturally. This isn't about forced restraint but a genuine lack of desire as your body adjusts to the nourishment provided by animal-based foods.

The Role of Health Considerations

1.   Addressing Specific Health Challenges

For individuals with conditions such as inflammation, autoimmune issues, or gut sensitivities, a stricter carnivore approach may be beneficial. Reducing or eliminating foods that trigger symptoms can lead to profound improvements in well-being.

2.   Flexibility for General Health

For those without pressing health concerns, the level of restriction can be more relaxed. Occasional indulgences or deviations won't derail your progress as long as they align with your overall sense of well-being.

The Natural Appeal of Animal-Based Foods

1.   Comfort and Satiation

Many find that animal-based foods naturally become their comfort foods. The richness of fatty cuts of beef, the savory satisfaction of pork sausages, and the delicate flavors of seafood provide both nourishment and emotional fulfillment.

2.   Diversity Within Animal Foods

A carnivore diet offers surprising variety:

• Large ruminants such as beef and lamb
• Pork products, from bacon to sausages
• Poultry, like chicken and turkey
• Seafood, including cold-water fish, shellfish, and smaller species
• Dairy and eggs, if tolerated

This diversity ensures that the diet remains enjoyable and sustainable over time.

The Importance of Fats and Oils

1.   Prioritizing Fats for Energy

Fats are essential in a carnivore diet, providing the primary source of energy. Fatty cuts of meat, animal-based oils, and cold-water fish are excellent options to ensure sufficient fat intake.

2.   Satiation and Taste

A higher fat content not only supports metabolic health but also enhances the flavor and satiation of meals, making it easier to maintain the lifestyle.

Voluntary Restrictions vs. Rules

1.   Empowering Choice

Restrictions in a carnivore diet should never feel like a burden. Instead, they are choices driven by personal experience and a desire for optimal health.

2.   Evolving Preferences

As you progress in your journey, your preferences and tolerance levels may shift. This natural evolution allows you to fine-tune your approach without rigid adherence to external rules.

Balance and Long-Term Sustainability

The most successful carnivore diets are those that prioritize balance and sustainability. Being overly rigid can lead to burnout, while being overly lenient can compromise results. Finding a middle ground that suits your lifestyle, goals, and biology ensures long-term success and satisfaction.

Empowering Individual Exploration

"How restrictive should I be?" is a question only you can answer. By embracing carnivore as a personal journey, guided by your body's signals and your evolving preferences, you can create a lifestyle that nurtures both health and happiness. Through experimentation and mindful choices, the carnivore diet becomes not a restriction but a path to greater freedom and vitality.

Blood Work: Expect Changes

Adopting a meat-centric diet as a carnivore fundamentally shifts your body's biochemistry and metabolism, which will naturally reflect in your blood work. These changes are not inherently harmful, but they often defy conventional medical expectations because most established markers are based on data from a population overwhelmingly composed of plant-based or mixed-diet eaters. Understanding these differences can help you interpret your health accurately and avoid unnecessary concern.

Lipid Panel: Challenging Conventional Wisdom

One of the most striking changes will likely occur in your lipid panel, particularly in cholesterol levels:

1.   Total Cholesterol and LDL

Carnivores often see an increase in total cholesterol and low-density lipoprotein (LDL). While traditionally considered a risk factor for heart disease, emerging research shows that higher cholesterol is associated with better longevity and reduced rates of neurodegenerative diseases. LDL plays critical roles in immune function and cellular repair, and its elevation in carnivores should be considered in this context.

2.   Triglycerides and HDL

On the flip side, triglycerides typically decrease significantly, and high-density lipoprotein (HDL), often called "good cholesterol," increases. This ratio—low triglycerides to high HDL—is a far better predictor of cardiovascular health than LDL alone and reflects the metabolic benefits of a carnivore lifestyle.

Blood Glucose and A1C: Interpreting the Anomalies

1.   Stable Blood Glucose

On a carnivore diet, blood glucose levels often stabilize at lower ranges due to the absence of carbohydrate spikes. However, glucose readings may occasionally appear higher than expected during fasting due to a process called gluconeogenesis, where your body produces glucose from protein for specific energy needs.

2.   Hemoglobin A1C

A1C measures the percentage of glycated hemoglobin, often used as a marker for average blood glucose levels over three months. In carnivores, this marker may rise slightly, not because of poor glucose control, but because red blood cells tend to live longer on a nutrient-dense, low-inflammatory diet. This extended lifespan can skew A1C upward.

Other Biomarkers

1.   Inflammatory Markers

Markers like C-reactive protein (CRP) and homocysteine often decrease, reflecting lower systemic inflammation.

2.   Uric Acid

Uric acid levels may rise temporarily as your body adapts, but this usually stabilizes over time. Elevated uric acid in the context of low inflammation and metabolic health is less concerning than previously thought.

3.   Thyroid Function

Thyroid hormone levels, particularly T3, may decrease. This does not necessarily indicate poor thyroid function but rather reflects improved energy efficiency and reduced metabolic stress due to lower systemic inflammation and a fat-based metabolism.

Context Matters: You're Not the Norm

The conventional reference ranges for blood work are based on a predominantly plant-eating population with mixed metabolic health. These ranges do not necessarily apply to carnivores, who represent a unique and under-studied cohort. Instead of comparing your results to the general population, consider the following:

1.   Seek a Specialist

Work with a healthcare provider experienced with carnivores or low-carb lifestyles who understands the nuances of your blood work.

2.   Track Trends Over Time

Rather than focusing on single readings, observe how your markers change over months and years. Consistency in health outcomes, such as energy, mental clarity, and physical performance, often matters more than isolated numbers.

Empower Yourself with Knowledge

1.   Learn the Science

Dive into the latest research on cholesterol, insulin resistance, and metabolic health to better understand the implications of your results. Resources such as the work of Dr. Paul Saladino or Dr. Ken Berry can offer valuable insights.

2.   Challenge Outdated Assumptions

Be prepared to question conventional advice and educate yourself on how metabolic health differs when carbohydrates are largely eliminated from your diet.

Advocate for Yourself

Doctors unfamiliar with the carnivore diet may express concern about your blood work. They are trained to flag deviations from the "normal" ranges without considering the context of a radically different dietary approach. You may need to respectfully advocate for yourself, providing explanations or even seeking second opinions from practitioners more aligned with your lifestyle.

Summary: Blood Work as a New Normal

Blood work as a carnivore reflects the profound biochemical shift that accompanies this lifestyle. While certain markers like cholesterol or A1C may trigger alarms in traditional medical paradigms, they often represent adaptations to a low-carb, fat-based metabolism rather than health risks. Understanding these changes and working with knowledgeable healthcare professionals will help you navigate these discussions with confidence and clarity.

> *Embrace the opportunity to redefine "normal" based on your vibrant health, not outdated metrics.*

Supplements - Fewer are needed.

Iodine remains under-appreciated.

One of the most profound shifts on a carnivore diet is the reduced need for supplements. When eating a plant-dominant diet, people often face challenges like malabsorption, nutrient deficiencies, and the intake of anti-nutrients (such as oxalates and phytates) that hinder mineral absorption and overall health.

However, iodine deficiency, soil depletion, and individual health conditions may necessitate targeted supplementation. Additionally, some choose to explore supplements that promote healthspan and longevity as an elective pursuit.

Why Fewer Supplements Are Needed

A carnivore diet reduces or eliminates the need for many common supplements by providing highly bioavailable nutrients and avoiding anti-nutrients that hinder absorption.

High-quality animal products inherently provides bioavailable forms of essential nutrients like iron, B vitamins (especially B12), zinc, and omega-3 fatty acids, significantly diminishing the reliance on supplements.

1.   Eliminating Anti-Nutrients

Plants contain substances like oxalates, phytates, and lectins that bind essential minerals and prevent their absorption. Removing these from the diet allows for more efficient nutrient uptake from food.

2.   Nutrient Density of Animal Foods

High-quality animal products are nutrient powerhouses, supplying nearly all the vitamins, minerals, and fatty acids humans need in their most bioavailable forms. For example:

- **Iron** is readily absorbed from red meat, unlike the less bioavailable form found in plants.
- **B12**, a critical nutrient absent in plants, is abundant in animal-based diets.
- **Omega-3 fatty acids**, essential for brain and heart health, are found in fatty fish and grass-fed meats.

3.   Reduced Metabolic Burden

With lower systemic inflammation and improved digestion on a meat-based diet, the body's efficiency in utilizing nutrients increases, reducing the perceived need for external supplementation.

Situations Where Supplements May Be Necessary

While many nutritional needs are met through carnivory, there are areas where supplementation may still serve a purpose:

1.   Specific Health Conditions or Genetic Variants

Individuals with certain genetic predispositions or health challenges may benefit from targeted supplementation. For example:

- **MTHFR** Gene Variants – People with impaired MTHFR function may require methylated folate or B12 for optimal methylation and detoxification.

- Autoimmune or Chronic Illness – Disease states may necessitate supplementation with vitamins or minerals that are otherwise difficult to obtain in sufficient quantities through diet alone.

2.   Iodine Deficiency

Iodine remains one of the most underappreciated nutrients. Modern agricultural practices have depleted iodine levels in soils, and even high-quality animal foods may not provide enough. Supplementing with iodine, such as through kelp tablets or iodine drops, can help support thyroid function and overall health.

3.   Soil Depletion

Although carnivory addresses many deficiencies, modern agricultural practices have reduced nutrient density in the food supply. This includes not only iodine but potentially selenium, magnesium, and other trace minerals.

4.   Exploration of Healthspan and Lifespan Substances

As longevity research advances, some people explore specialty supplements to enhance healthspan. These might include:

- **Collagen** or **Glycine** to support connective tissue, skin, and joint health.
- **Creatine** for enhanced muscle function and cognitive benefits.
- **NMN** or **Resveratrol** for potential anti-aging effects.

Benefits of Strategic Supplementation

Carnivores may not need routine supplementation, but targeted approaches can offer benefits:

1.　　Preventive Health

Supplements like iodine or magnesium may fill gaps that even high-quality animal foods cannot address due to environmental factors.

2.　　Optimizing Performance

Supplements like creatine or taurine can enhance physical and mental performance.

3.　　Experimentation with Longevity

Exploring cutting-edge compounds may offer opportunities to extend healthspan and vitality.

Approaching Supplements with Intention

The key to supplement use on a carnivore diet is intentionality:

- *Assess Your Needs:* Understand your specific health context, including any genetic or medical predispositions, before starting supplements.
- *Test and Measure:* Use blood tests and other diagnostics to identify deficiencies or imbalances that may benefit from supplementation.
- *Start Simple:* Begin with basic, well-studied supplements like iodine or magnesium if needed, and observe how your body responds.

Conclusion: The Minimalist Approach to Supplements

Ultimately, the goal is not to reject supplements entirely but to use them purposefully and as complements to the nutrient-dense foundation of a carnivore diet.

Has it gotten warmer?

One fascinating and often surprising change for many who adopt the Carnivore diet is an increased tolerance for colder conditions. You may notice that environments or temperatures that previously felt chilly now feel comfortably warm. This phenomenon often raises questions, and understanding it involves a deeper look at how the Carnivore diet impacts metabolism, circulation, and overall thermoregulation.

Why Does This Happen?

1.   Increased Metabolic Rate

Nutrient-Dense Foods: The Carnivore diet provides a constant supply of highly bioavailable nutrients, including essential fats and proteins. These fuel your body efficiently, often increasing your basal metabolic rate.

Fat Oxidation: When your body relies on fat as its primary fuel source, it generates more stable and sustained energy, which can contribute to a feeling of warmth.

2.   Improved Circulation

A reduction in inflammation may improve circulation, allowing blood to flow more efficiently to extremities and maintaining warmth even in cooler conditions.

3.   Stable Blood Sugar Levels

By eliminating carbohydrate spikes and crashes, the Carnivore diet stabilizes blood sugar levels. This helps prevent the sudden chills often associated with low blood sugar or energy crashes.

4.   Thermogenesis

Eating high-protein foods promotes thermogenesis—the process by which your body generates heat during digestion. This may contribute to the feeling of increased warmth after meals.

The Subjective Experience

1.   Temperature Tolerance

- You may find yourself needing fewer layers in colder weather or feeling less reliant on external heat sources, such as heaters or blankets.
- Activities like walking in brisk weather or sleeping in a cooler room may become more comfortable.

2.   Warmth After Meals

Consuming a protein-heavy, fatty meal often results in a pleasant feeling of warmth as your body digests and metabolizes the nutrients.

3.   Mental Clarity and Energy Connection

The improved energy levels and mental clarity associated with Carnivore can make you less aware of cold discomfort, as your body functions more efficiently overall.

Practical Implications

1.   Adjusting Your Environment

- You might need to reconsider your typical approach to dressing for the weather. Layers you once thought essential might now feel unnecessary.
- You may reduce energy use for heating, contributing to cost savings and environmental benefits.

2.   Seasonal Activities

Colder outdoor activities that previously felt daunting—like winter hikes or chilly morning walks—may now feel enjoyable.

3.   Social Perceptions

Others might comment on how lightly dressed you are for the weather or wonder why you don't seem cold. Be prepared to explain (if you wish) or simply smile and enjoy your newfound warmth.

4. Possible Caveats

1.   Too Warm?

In rare cases, some individuals might feel uncomfortably warm or experience increased sweating. This could indicate that your metabolism is running high, and adjusting fat or protein intake might help.

2.   Not Universal

This effect may vary between individuals, depending on factors such as metabolic health, activity level, and baseline body composition.

Broader Context

1.   Connection to Other Benefits

This newfound warmth ties into the broader metabolic and systemic improvements seen on Carnivore. Your body is functioning as intended, processing food efficiently and reducing unnecessary energy loss.

2.   Evolutionary Perspective

A diet focused on nutrient-dense, animal-based foods aligns with our evolutionary history, which may explain this effect. Early humans relied on fat and protein to maintain energy and warmth in colder climates, supporting the idea that this warmth is a return to a more natural state.

6. Conclusion

The feeling that "it has gotten warmer" is one of the many subtle yet profound changes brought about by the Carnivore diet.

> *This warmth is a reflection of your body operating more efficiently, with improved metabolism, stable energy, and reduced inflammation. Embrace it as a sign that your dietary choices are positively influencing your overall well-being.*

As a Carnivore, You Are Not Representative of "Normal"

The truth is, normal is defined by the majority, and as a carnivore, you stand apart from that majority. In today's world, a meat-first diet makes you a small minority, and this carries profound implications for how your health, choices, and even worldview are perceived.

Medical Norms Are Skewed

The benchmarks of "normal" in medical practice—be it lab test ranges, dietary recommendations, or health markers—are all based on populations that predominantly consume a mix of plant and animal foods. Many of these diets are heavily skewed toward processed and plant-based options. The result is a baseline that reflects a population often grappling with chronic disease, metabolic dysfunction, and nutrient deficiencies. As a carnivore, your unique physiology may fall outside these established norms.

For example, you may encounter:

Unusual Lab Results: Elevated cholesterol levels, which are normal for a carnivore and can correlate with longevity, might be flagged as dangerous.

Dietary Skepticism: Professionals may view your diet as extreme or unbalanced simply because it doesn't align with conventional guidelines.

The Plant-Based Narrative Dominates

The cultural zeitgeist is saturated with the message that plant-based diets are healthier, more ethical, and environmentally superior. This narrative dominates public discourse, medical advice, and health research. Many studies on diet are observational, rife with confounding variables, and shaped by the prevailing biases of researchers and funding sources—often tied to industries that benefit from processed foods and pharmaceuticals.

For carnivores, this means navigating a landscape where the majority of dietary advice is irrelevant, misleading, or even harmful.

The Importance of N=1 Science

Since the carnivore lifestyle isn't widely studied or represented in scientific literature, personal experimentation—what's often called "N=1" science—becomes crucial. Anecdotal evidence, while dismissed by some, is a vital source of insight in this realm. Your own body becomes the laboratory, and you learn to trust your experiences, results, and intuition over generalized recommendations.

Connect With the Community

Fortunately, you are not alone. The carnivore community is vibrant and growing, with many advocates sharing their journeys, experiences, and insights online. Platforms like YouTube, forums, and social media offer a wealth of support, inspiration, and practical advice. Engaging with others who understand your perspective can be a lifeline when the world around you seems to misunderstand or reject your choices.

Embrace Your Uniqueness

Being outside the norm isn't a flaw—it's a strength. Carnivores are charting new territory, questioning old assumptions, and demonstrating what's possible with a diet rooted in ancestral wisdom and modern determination. By stepping away from the "normal" that often correlates with unhealth, you're aligning with vitality, resilience, and independence.

> *So, wear your difference proudly. Normal isn't always healthy, and being part of a minority often means you're ahead of the curve.*

Tracking Your Progress

Progress on a carnivore diet can be as rewarding as it is complex, but it requires establishing a baseline and knowing what to look for. Progress, after all, is measured against expectations — whether subjective (how you feel) or objective (what you can measure). Let's explore these two key dimensions and how they interplay in tracking your journey.

Subjective Metrics: How Do You Feel?

Subjective measures are often the most immediate and motivating indicators of progress. They include:

Energy Levels: Do you feel a sustained energy throughout the day, free from the mid-afternoon slump?

Wakefulness: Are you waking up feeling refreshed and ready to engage with the day?

Mental Clarity: Are you experiencing sharper thinking and reduced mental fog?

Gusto for Life: Do you feel enthusiasm for tasks and an increased sense of vitality?

Absence of Dysfunction: Are common issues like headaches, bloating, or joint pain reduced or eliminated?

These metrics can vary daily and even hourly, making it essential to tune into patterns rather than isolated moments. A journal can be a valuable tool for tracking your subjective experience over time.

Objective Metrics: What Can You Measure?

While subjective experiences provide insight, objective data offers tangible evidence of your body's response to a carnivore diet.

1.   Ketones

- Why Measure? The presence of ketones indicates your body is using fat as its primary energy source, a hallmark of nutritional ketosis.
- How? Using a breath analyzer to measure acetone is a convenient and non-invasive way to monitor ketones. Consistently elevated acetone levels suggest effective fat metabolism.

2.   Blood Glucose

- Why Measure? Stable blood glucose levels indicate metabolic flexibility and reduced reliance on carbohydrates for energy.
- How? A CGM (Continuous Glucose Monitor) offers real-time feedback on blood sugar trends. Look for:
- Morning Glucose Rises: A natural phenomenon called the dawn effect, where your liver produces glucose (via gluconeogenesis) to kickstart your day.
- Post-Meal Stability: Ideally, your blood glucose remains steady without significant spikes, even after eating.

3.   Other Biomarkers

If you wish to dive deeper, consider periodic lab tests to monitor markers like triglycerides, HDL/LDL cholesterol, and inflammatory markers (like CRP). These can provide additional insights into the long-term effects of your diet.

The Balance Between Subjective and Objective

Both subjective and objective metrics are valuable, but they must be interpreted together. For example:

- A day of low energy (subjective) might correspond with lower ketone readings (objective), prompting you to examine your fat intake or sleep quality.
- Stable blood glucose readings (objective) paired with mental clarity and enthusiasm (subjective) affirm you're on the right path.

The Role of Expectations

Tracking progress also means aligning your expectations with reality. Understand that:

- *Progress isn't always linear.* Some days may feel like a step backward, but they can be part of a broader trend of improvement.
- *Your goals might shift.* What begins as a focus on weight loss might evolve into prioritizing mental clarity or athletic performance.

Tips for Effective Tracking

- *Be Consistent*: Measure at the same time daily (e.g., blood glucose in the morning, ketones mid-afternoon).
- *Use a Journal*: Document both subjective feelings and objective data to observe trends over weeks, not just days.
- *Experiment Intentionally*: Adjust one variable at a time (e.g., increasing fat intake or tweaking fasting windows) to assess its impact on your metrics.

- ***Focus on the Big Picture***: A single bad day doesn't mean failure. Look for overall trends and long-term patterns.

Tracking your progress on a carnivore diet is as much an art as it is a science. By combining how you feel with what you can measure, you can fine-tune your approach, celebrate your wins, and address any challenges along the way.

> *The ultimate goal isn't just to collect data—it's to empower yourself to make informed decisions that align with your health and lifestyle aspirations.*

N=1 Science: The Call of Personal Experimentation

In the context of the Carnivore lifestyle, "N=1" refers to experiments conducted on a single subject—you. Unlike traditional scientific studies that analyze data from large groups, N=1 experiments focus on personal observations and outcomes, recognizing that what works for one person may not work for another.

This approach aligns with the Grand Dilemma's core challenge: the need to navigate a unique path in a world structured around generalized dietary norms. By conducting N=1 experiments, you take ownership of your health, tailoring your lifestyle based on direct experience rather than relying solely on external guidelines or societal expectations.

Key elements of N=1 experimentation include:

Observation and Tracking: Monitor your body's responses to dietary changes, new foods, fasting protocols, or reintroductions. Tools like journals, continuous glucose monitors, or ketone meters can provide valuable insights.

Adaptation and Learning: Use your findings to refine your choices. Whether it's eliminating a trigger food or optimizing your fat-to-protein ratio, the goal is continuous improvement.

Patience and Consistency: Results often take time. Allow your body to adjust to changes and maintain consistency to accurately evaluate outcomes.

Transgressions Become More Painful

Adapting to a carnivore diet often transforms how we experience and respond to food. Many carnivores report that indulging in plant-based foods after becoming fully adapted to a meat-first lifestyle leads to pronounced physical and mental distress. This phenomenon can feel deeply frustrating, especially when it disrupts cherished traditions or cravings for once-enjoyable meals.

The Experience of Transgressions

What many call a "transgression"—eating a conventional meal with plant-based ingredients—can trigger:

- *Digestive Distress:* Stomach pain, bloating, gas, or diarrhea.
- *Inflammatory Symptoms:* Red, itchy, or watery eyes; sneezing; runny nose; or even skin rashes.
- *Neurological Effects:* Brain fog, headaches, dizziness, or disorientation.
- *General Malaise:* Fatigue, irritability, or a sense of being "off."

These reactions can be surprising, especially if you once ate such meals regularly with seemingly no ill effects.

Why Didn't This Happen Before?

Prior to adopting a carnivore diet, your body may have been in a state of chronic adaptation to dietary stressors. Over time, many of us become desensitized to the effects of plant-based foods or processed meals, which may contribute to the accumulation of underlying metabolic disorders. However, when we remove these stressors and allow our bodies to heal:

1.   Clearing Out Toxins

Many plant foods contain anti-nutrients and toxins (e.g., oxalates, lectins) that can accumulate in the body. Over time on a carnivore diet, these compounds are eliminated, and the body resets. When you reintroduce these toxins, the body responds with heightened sensitivity —what you now feel might have been happening subtly all along.

2.   Reduced Inflammation

The chronic low-grade inflammation you may have carried while eating a mixed diet gets resolved on carnivore. With your baseline inflammation lower, even small exposures to inflammatory foods stand out dramatically.

3.   Recalibrated Immune System

A healed gut and restored immune function can overreact to plant-based foods it now recognizes as irritants, amplifying symptoms.

4.   Increased Awareness

On carnivore, you likely feel clearer, lighter, and more energetic. Returning to plant-based foods creates a stark contrast, making discomfort impossible to ignore.

The Disappointment of Fond Memories

Many of us have emotional or cultural attachments to certain foods. A grandmother's casserole, holiday treats, or beloved ethnic dishes might hold sentimental value. The realization that these foods now cause discomfort can feel like a betrayal of cherished traditions or connections.

This disappointment is compounded by a sense of loss — not just of the food, but of the social and cultural moments tied to it.

Reframing Transgressions

Rather than viewing these reactions as setbacks, you might consider them insights:

1.   A Clear Message from Your Body

Your body is now more honest about how it reacts to certain foods. What once seemed "normal" was likely a constant state of low-level dysfunction.

2.   A Tool for Refinement

These responses can help you identify specific foods or ingredients that are most problematic, empowering you to make informed choices.

3.   A Reminder of Progress

The dramatic reactions to transgressions highlight just how far you've come in improving your health and well-being.

Strategies for Managing Transgressions

1.   Be Selective

If you choose to indulge, make it meaningful. Opt for foods that hold the most emotional or cultural value, and avoid mindless deviations.

2.   Prepare Your Body

Some find that easing into transgressions—eating small amounts or pairing them with fat—can reduce the intensity of reactions.

3.   Embrace Alternatives

Explore carnivore-friendly ways to recreate cherished dishes. For example, substitute cauliflower for rice or make a meat-based version of a favorite recipe.

4.   Lean on Community

Sharing your experiences with other carnivores can provide validation and support, reminding you that you're not alone in navigating these challenges.

Final Thoughts

Experiencing the discomfort of transgressions isn't a failure—it's a testament to the healing power of the carnivore lifestyle. While it can feel disappointing to lose the ability to eat certain foods without consequence, it's also an opportunity to embrace a deeper awareness of your body's needs.

> *In time, you may find that the clarity, vitality, and well-being you gain on carnivore far outweigh the temporary pleasures of old dietary habits.*

A small BIT OF METABOLIC SCIENCE

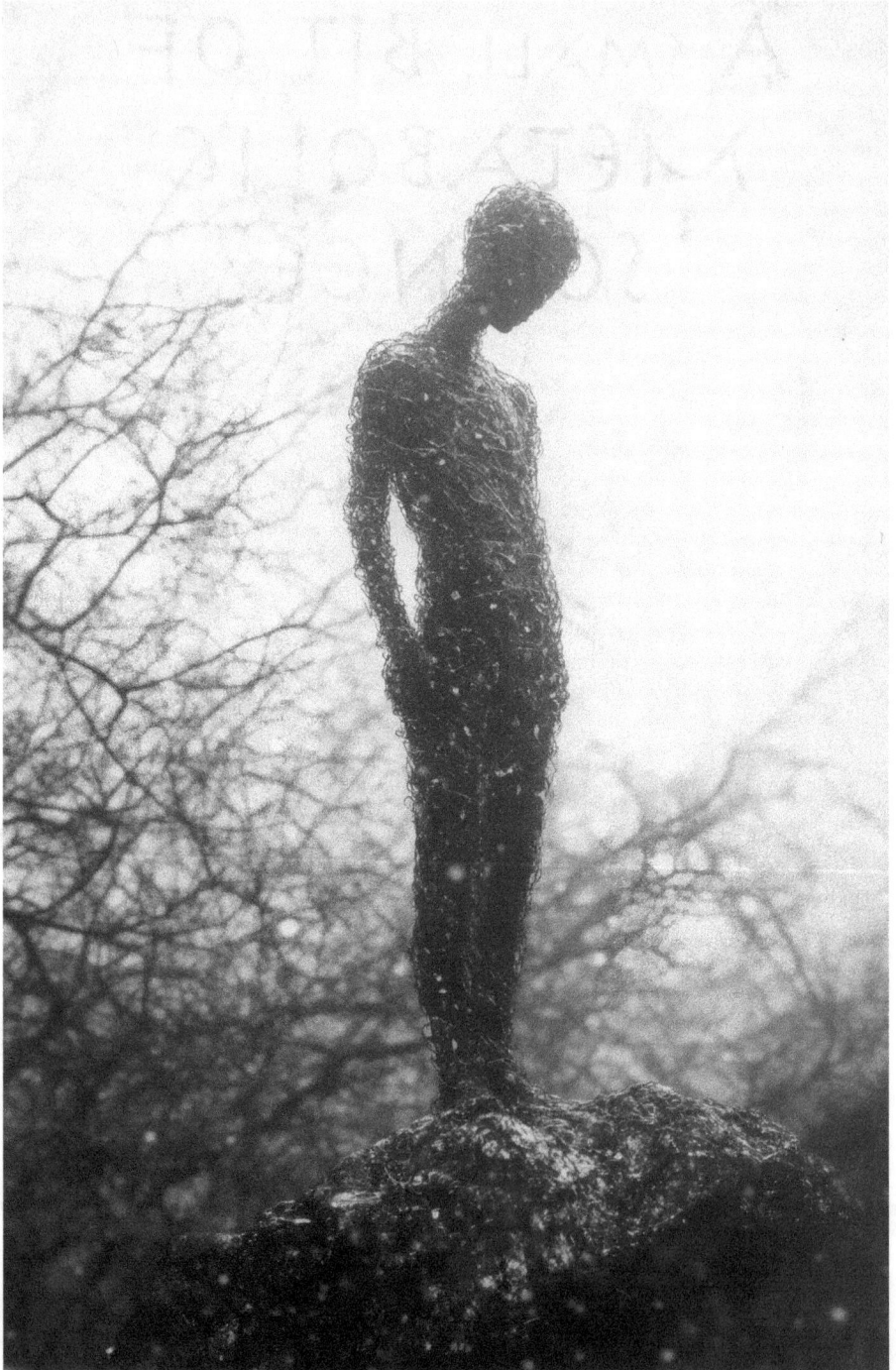

Overview of Glucose Metabolism

Glucose metabolism is the process by which the body uses glucose—a simple sugar and primary energy source for many tissues—to produce energy in the form of adenosine triphosphate (ATP). It involves several interconnected pathways that allow cells to extract energy efficiently, store it for later use, or produce metabolic intermediates for other cellular processes.

1. Key Steps in Glucose Metabolism

a. Glycolysis

- Location: Cytoplasm
- Process: Glucose (6-carbon molecule) is broken down into two molecules of pyruvate (3-carbon molecule).
- ATP Yield: Produces a net gain of 2 ATP molecules and 2 NADH (electron carriers).
- Significance: Glycolysis does not require oxygen, making it an anaerobic pathway.

b. Pyruvate Pathways

- In the presence of oxygen, pyruvate enters the mitochondria for further breakdown (aerobic respiration).
- Without oxygen, pyruvate is converted into lactate in the cytoplasm (anaerobic metabolism), a process that allows glycolysis to continue by regenerating NAD+.

c. Citric Acid Cycle (Krebs Cycle)

- Location: Mitochondria
- Process: Pyruvate is converted into acetyl-CoA, which enters the cycle. The cycle generates electron carriers (NADH, FADH2) and releases carbon dioxide as a byproduct.
- ATP Yield: Minimal direct ATP production, but significant generation of reducing equivalents for the electron transport chain.

d. Electron Transport Chain (ETC) and Oxidative Phosphorylation

- Location: Inner mitochondrial membrane
- Process: NADH and FADH2 donate electrons to the ETC, creating a proton gradient across the mitochondrial membrane. The flow of protons back into the mitochondria through ATP synthase drives ATP production.
- ATP Yield: Approximately 32-34 ATP per molecule of glucose.

2. Glucose Storage and Release

a. Glycogenesis

- Process: Excess glucose is stored as glycogen in the liver and muscles.
- Significance: Glycogen provides a quick source of glucose during short-term fasting or intense exercise.

b. Glycogenolysis

- Process: Glycogen is broken down into glucose-6-phosphate for energy production or free glucose (in the liver) to maintain blood sugar levels.

c. Gluconeogenesis

- Process: The liver (and kidneys, to a lesser extent) synthesizes glucose from non-carbohydrate sources, such as lactate, glycerol, and amino acids, to maintain blood sugar levels during prolonged fasting or carbohydrate restriction.

3. Hormonal Regulation

- Insulin: Promotes glucose uptake into cells, glycolysis, and glycogenesis while inhibiting gluconeogenesis and glycogenolysis.
- Glucagon: Opposes insulin by stimulating glycogenolysis and gluconeogenesis during fasting states.
- Other Hormones: Epinephrine, cortisol, and growth hormone also modulate glucose metabolism during stress, fasting, or exercise.

4. Metabolic Flexibility

While glucose is a primary energy source, the body can switch to alternative fuels, such as fatty acids and ketones, during periods of fasting, carbohydrate restriction, or prolonged exercise. This shift reduces dependence on glucose and preserves glycogen for critical functions like brain activity.

5. Relevance to Health

Efficient glucose metabolism is crucial for energy balance and overall health. Dysregulation, such as insulin resistance or chronic hyperglycemia, contributes to metabolic disorders like Type 2 diabetes, obesity, and cardiovascular disease.

Understanding glucose metabolism provides insights into dietary strategies, exercise, and therapeutic interventions to optimize energy use and maintain metabolic health.

Overview of Fat Metabolism

Fat metabolism refers to the processes by which the body breaks down fats (lipids) to produce energy and synthesizes or stores fats for future use. Fats are a dense and efficient energy source, yielding more than twice the energy per gram compared to carbohydrates or proteins. The primary pathways of fat metabolism include lipolysis, beta-oxidation, and lipid storage.

1. Key Components of Fat Metabolism

a. Types of Fats in the Body

- Triglycerides: Stored in adipose tissue and muscles, they are the main energy reserve.
- Free Fatty Acids (FFAs): Released from triglycerides during lipolysis.
- Cholesterol: Used in cell membranes and as a precursor for steroid hormones and bile acids.
- Phospholipids: Essential for cell membrane structure and signaling.

b. Key Sources of Fats

- Dietary Fats: Consumed from foods, including saturated fats, monounsaturated fats, polyunsaturated fats, and cholesterol.
- Stored Fats: Body fat reserves in adipose tissue.

2. Key Steps in Fat Metabolism

a. Lipolysis

- Process: Triglycerides stored in adipose tissue are broken down into glycerol and free fatty acids (FFAs).
- Enzymes: Hormone-sensitive lipase (HSL) and lipoprotein lipase (LPL).
- Triggers: Stimulated by hormones like epinephrine, norepinephrine, and glucagon during fasting, exercise, or stress.

b. Transport of Free Fatty Acids

- FFAs are released into the bloodstream and bind to albumin for transport to tissues requiring energy.

c. Beta-Oxidation

- Location: Mitochondria
- Process: FFAs are broken down into two-carbon units of acetyl-CoA.
- Products: Acetyl-CoA, NADH, and FADH2, which feed into the Krebs cycle and electron transport chain.
- Energy Yield: Fatty acids produce significantly more ATP compared to glucose. For example, the breakdown of palmitic acid (a 16-carbon fatty acid) yields 106 ATP molecules.

d. Ketogenesis

- Location: Liver
- Process: Excess acetyl-CoA from beta-oxidation is converted into ketone bodies (e.g., beta-hydroxybutyrate, acetoacetate, acetone).

- Purpose: Ketones provide an alternative energy source for the brain, heart, and muscles during prolonged fasting, carbohydrate restriction, or ketogenic diets.

e. Lipogenesis

- Process: Excess dietary carbohydrates and fats are converted into triglycerides and stored in adipose tissue.
- Location: Mainly in the liver and adipose tissue.

3. Regulation of Fat Metabolism

Hormonal Regulation

- Insulin: Inhibits lipolysis and promotes fat storage (lipogenesis).
- Glucagon: Stimulates lipolysis and fat mobilization.
- Epinephrine and Norepinephrine: Activate hormone-sensitive lipase, promoting lipolysis during stress or exercise.
- Leptin: Regulates energy balance by signaling satiety and influencing fat storage.

4. Metabolic Advantages of Fat

- Energy Density: Fats provide 9 calories per gram compared to 4 calories per gram for carbohydrates and proteins.
- Storage Efficiency: Fat is stored with minimal water, making it a lightweight, long-term energy reserve.
- Sustained Energy: Fat metabolism provides steady energy for prolonged activities, unlike glucose, which is rapidly depleted.

5. Clinical and Health Relevance

a. Importance in Low-Carbohydrate and Ketogenic Diets

- Fat becomes the primary fuel source when carbohydrate intake is low.
- Ketone production provides energy for the brain, especially during fasting or carbohydrate restriction.

b. Dysregulation of Fat Metabolism

- Obesity: Excess fat storage due to an energy surplus.
- Insulin Resistance: Impaired regulation of fat and glucose metabolism.
- Hyperlipidemia: High levels of circulating triglycerides and cholesterol, associated with cardiovascular disease.

6. Interplay Between Fat and Glucose Metabolism

The Randall Cycle highlights the competition between fat and carbohydrate metabolism for energy production. When one is dominant, it inhibits the other. This metabolic flexibility ensures that the body optimizes energy use based on availability.

Conclusion

Fat metabolism is a cornerstone of human energy systems, offering efficient energy storage and production. Its regulation by hormonal and metabolic signals ensures that the body adapts to varying energy demands, making it essential for survival and optimal health. Understanding fat metabolism is crucial for managing energy balance, weight, and overall metabolic health.

Overview of Carbohydrate Metabolism

Carbohydrates are a broad category of macronutrients that include sugars, starches, and fibers. They serve primarily as a source of glucose, the body's most readily available fuel. When consumed, carbohydrates undergo a multi-step process of digestion, absorption, and metabolism, leading to the production of energy in the form of ATP (adenosine triphosphate). However, their effects on blood glucose levels and overall metabolism depend on the type of carbohydrate consumed.

Types of Carbohydrates

1.   Simple Sugars (Monosaccharides and Disaccharides)

Monosaccharides: Glucose, fructose, and galactose. These are the basic units of carbohydrates and are absorbed directly into the bloodstream.

Disaccharides: Sucrose (glucose + fructose), lactose (glucose + galactose), and maltose (two glucose molecules). These need to be broken down into monosaccharides before absorption.

2.   Complex Carbohydrates (Polysaccharides)

Long chains of glucose molecules, found in starches (like grains, potatoes, and legumes) and fibers.

Starches are readily broken down into glucose, while fibers are indigestible and have minimal impact on blood glucose.

Digestion and Absorption

1.   Simple Sugars

Sucrose: Broken down into glucose and fructose by the enzyme sucrase in the small intestine.

Fructose: Absorbed separately and metabolized primarily in the liver, where it can be converted to glucose, glycogen, or fat.

The breakdown and absorption of sucrose are slower than that of pure glucose due to the need for enzymatic cleavage.

2.   Complex Carbohydrates

Starch: Digested rapidly by amylase enzymes in the saliva and pancreas into maltose and then into free glucose molecules.

The "unzipping" of glucose from starches can lead to a significant and rapid spike in blood glucose levels, often more pronounced than from sucrose consumption.

Metabolism

1.   Glucose Utilization

Once absorbed, glucose enters the bloodstream, leading to a rise in blood sugar levels.

Insulin is released by the pancreas to facilitate glucose uptake by cells for immediate energy or storage as glycogen in the liver and muscles.

Any excess glucose is converted to fat through lipogenesis when glycogen stores are full.

2.   Fructose Metabolism

Fructose is transported to the liver, where it bypasses regulatory steps in glucose metabolism.

Excess fructose can contribute to fat production and storage, potentially leading to non-alcoholic fatty liver disease (NAFLD) with chronic overconsumption.

3.   Glycemic Response

Foods high in simple sugars or starches with minimal fiber cause rapid spikes in blood glucose levels.

This can lead to insulin spikes, subsequent crashes in blood sugar, and cycles of hunger and energy fluctuations.

The Problem with Rapid Digestion

The body's ability to quickly digest starches into glucose means that certain carbohydrate-rich foods (like white bread, rice, or potatoes) can have a glycemic impact similar to or greater than pure sugar. These spikes and crashes can strain metabolic pathways over time, potentially leading to insulin resistance, weight gain, and type 2 diabetes.

Key Differences: Sucrose vs. Starch

Sucrose: Requires enzymatic cleavage into glucose and fructose, slowing the immediate blood glucose impact.

Starch: Quickly "unzips" into pure glucose, causing rapid and significant increases in blood sugar, which can be more metabolically challenging.

Understanding these processes highlights why the type of carbohydrate matters just as much as the amount.

> *In a meat-centric or low-carb lifestyle, minimizing carbohydrate intake helps avoid these rapid glycemic fluctuations, promoting metabolic stability and fat-based energy production.*

Overview of Calories

The phrase "A calorie is not a calorie" challenges the simplistic idea that all calories are metabolically equivalent, emphasizing the differences in how the body processes energy from various macronutrients. While a calorie measures energy as a unit (1 calorie = 4.184 joules), the metabolic pathways that convert this energy into usable forms (e.g., ATP) vary significantly depending on the source—carbohydrate, fat, or protein. This concept underscores how the source of the calorie affects energy efficiency, biochemical impacts, and physiological outcomes.

Differences in ATP Yield: Glucose vs. Lipids

1. Glucose Metabolism (Carbohydrates)

- Pathway: Cellular glucose is metabolized primarily through glycolysis, the Krebs cycle, and the electron transport chain (ETC).
- ATP Yield:
- Glycolysis: 2 ATP (net) + 2 NADH (6 ATP after ETC).
- Pyruvate Oxidation: 2 NADH = 6 ATP.
- Krebs Cycle: 2 ATP + 6 NADH (18 ATP) + 2 FADH2 (4 ATP).
- Total ATP from One Molecule of Glucose: ~36–38 ATP.
- Caloric Energy Yield: 4 kcal/gram.
- Efficiency: Glucose is processed relatively quickly and primarily supports short-term, high-intensity activities.

2. Fat Metabolism (Lipids)

- Pathway: Fats are metabolized through lipolysis, beta-oxidation, the Krebs cycle, and the electron transport chain.
- ATP Yield: Significantly higher than glucose, due to the longer carbon chains in fatty acids:
- Example: Palmitic Acid (16-carbon fatty acid):
- Beta-oxidation: 7 NADH (21 ATP), 7 FADH2 (14 ATP), and 8 Acetyl-CoA.
- Acetyl-CoA (via Krebs): 24 NADH (72 ATP) + 8 FADH2 (16 ATP) + 8 GTP (8 ATP).
- Total ATP from One Palmitic Acid Molecule: ~106 ATP.
- Caloric Energy Yield: 9 kcal/gram.
- Efficiency: Fat provides a slow, steady energy supply, making it ideal for long-duration, low-intensity activities.

Key Differences Between Glucose and Fat Metabolism

a. Energy Density

Lipids provide over twice the energy (9 kcal/gram) compared to carbohydrates (4 kcal/gram). This makes fats more efficient for energy storage and prolonged energy release.

b. ATP Yield per Carbon Atom

Fats generate more ATP per carbon atom because their molecules are more reduced (contain more hydrogen), which yields more electrons for the ETC. For example:

- Glucose: ~6 ATP per carbon atom.
- Fatty acids: ~8 ATP per carbon atom.

c. Insulin Response

Carbohydrates stimulate a significant insulin response, promoting fat storage and suppressing fat mobilization.

Fats do not spike insulin, allowing the body to access fat stores more easily during fasting or ketogenic states.

d. Speed of Energy Production

Glucose metabolism is faster and supports rapid, immediate energy needs (e.g., sprinting).

Fat metabolism is slower and supports sustained energy over longer periods (e.g., endurance exercise).

Physiological Implications of ATP Yield Differences

Satiety and Energy Stability:

- Fat's high ATP yield and slower metabolism contribute to sustained energy levels and prolonged satiety.
- Glucose burns quickly, often leading to energy spikes followed by crashes.

Metabolic Flexibility:

- Carbohydrates are preferred during high-intensity activities because they are metabolized quickly.

- Fats are utilized during low-intensity or fasting states due to their efficiency and abundance.

Impact on Weight Management:

- Excess carbohydrates are readily converted to fat, while dietary fats are metabolized directly or stored efficiently.
- The energy cost of converting glucose into fat (de novo lipogenesis) is lower than the energy cost of oxidizing stored fat, favoring fat accumulation on high-carb diets.

Health Outcomes:

- Chronic reliance on glucose (and high insulin levels) is associated with metabolic issues like insulin resistance, obesity, and diabetes.
- Fat metabolism supports a ketogenic state, which can promote fat loss, improved insulin sensitivity, and mental clarity.

Conclusion

While the calorie is a standard unit of energy, the body processes calories from glucose and lipids very differently. Lipids provide a higher ATP yield per gram and per carbon atom, making them a more efficient and stable energy source. Understanding these differences is critical for tailoring diets to specific health goals, activity levels, and metabolic states. "A calorie is not a calorie" captures the nuanced interplay of biochemistry, metabolism, and physiology that goes beyond simple energy counting.

Overview of Cholesterol

Cholesterol is a waxy, fat-like substance that plays a vital role in the body. Despite its reputation as something to be avoided, cholesterol is essential for life. It is a structural component of every cell membrane, a precursor for hormone production, and a key player in the synthesis of vitamin D and bile acids, which help digest fats.

The body produces the majority of the cholesterol it needs, with the liver being the primary site of production. Dietary cholesterol, found in animal-based foods such as meat, eggs, and dairy, contributes only a fraction to the total cholesterol in the bloodstream for most individuals.

Cholesterol and Lipoproteins

Cholesterol travels through the bloodstream in particles called *lipoproteins*, which are categorized by their density:

Low-Density Lipoprotein (LDL): Often referred to as "bad cholesterol," LDL transports cholesterol from the liver to cells. High levels of LDL, especially small, dense particles, have been associated with an increased risk of cardiovascular disease (CVD). However, this relationship is complex and not solely determined by LDL levels.

High-Density Lipoprotein (HDL): Known as "good cholesterol," HDL carries cholesterol away from the bloodstream and back to the liver for processing or excretion. Higher HDL levels are typically associated with a reduced risk of CVD.

Triglycerides: Although not cholesterol, these fats are often measured alongside cholesterol. Elevated triglycerides can increase CVD risk, particularly when combined with low HDL and high LDL levels.

Cholesterol Myths and Misconceptions

For decades, dietary cholesterol was vilified for its supposed role in raising blood cholesterol and increasing heart disease risk. However, more recent research has revealed that for most people, dietary cholesterol has little impact on blood cholesterol levels. Instead, the body adjusts its cholesterol production based on dietary intake.

Cholesterol and Health

Hormones: Cholesterol is the building block for steroid hormones, including testosterone, estrogen, progesterone, and cortisol. Without adequate cholesterol, hormone production may suffer.

Cell Membranes: Cholesterol provides structural integrity and fluidity to cell membranes, enabling proper cell function and communication.

Brain and Nervous System: Cholesterol is abundant in the brain, where it is critical for neuronal function, synapse formation, and myelin sheath production.

Understanding Cholesterol in the Carnivore Context

> *For individuals on a carnivore diet, changes in blood*
> *cholesterol are common.*

Some people experience higher LDL and total cholesterol levels, often alongside improvements in HDL and triglycerides. While these changes can raise concerns, it's important to look beyond the traditional lipid panel and consider other markers of metabolic health, such as fasting insulin, HbA1c, and inflammatory markers like C-reactive protein (CRP).

Key Takeaways

- Cholesterol is not inherently "good" or "bad" but a critical component of human physiology.
- Context matters—elevated cholesterol in the presence of metabolic health and low inflammation may not carry the same risks as elevated cholesterol with poor metabolic health.
- Understanding cholesterol requires a holistic approach, focusing on overall health rather than isolated numbers.

If you're following a meat-first lifestyle, working with a healthcare provider who understands the nuances of cholesterol and metabolic health can help you navigate this complex topic confidently.

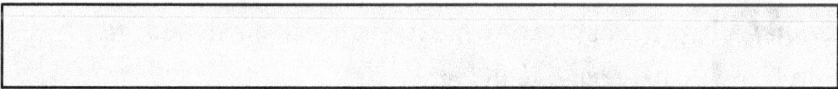

Overview of Ketones and Ketosis

Ketones are molecules produced by the liver during periods of low carbohydrate availability. They are an alternative fuel source, particularly for the brain and other energy-demanding tissues, when glucose is scarce. Ketones are derived from the breakdown of fats and serve as a vital metabolic adaptation that allows humans to survive and thrive during times of fasting, carbohydrate restriction, or high physical demand.

Ketosis is the metabolic state in which the body primarily uses ketones for energy instead of glucose. This state occurs when carbohydrate intake is sufficiently low to reduce insulin levels, signaling the body to shift its energy production from glucose to fats.

What Are Ketones?

Ketones are classified as ketone bodies, of which there are three primary types:

Beta-Hydroxybutyrate (BHB): The most abundant and energy-efficient ketone body.

Acetoacetate (AcAc): The precursor to BHB, which is also used directly as fuel.

Acetone: A byproduct of AcAc breakdown, often exhaled, giving the "fruity" breath associated with ketosis.

How Ketones Are Produced

Carbohydrate Restriction: When carb intake is low, glycogen stores in the liver are depleted, reducing glucose availability.

Fat Mobilization: The body begins to break down stored fat into fatty acids.

Ketogenesis: Fatty acids are transported to the liver, where they are converted into ketones.

Benefits of Ketosis

Ketosis is more than just a survival mechanism; it offers several physiological benefits:

- Stable Energy Levels: Ketones provide a slow-burning, consistent energy source, reducing energy crashes and hunger.
- Brain Fuel: Ketones cross the blood-brain barrier, supplying the brain with energy during low glucose availability. Many people report improved mental clarity and focus.
- Fat Burning: In ketosis, the body becomes highly efficient at mobilizing and oxidizing fat for energy.
- Reduced Inflammation: Ketones have anti-inflammatory properties, potentially benefiting conditions like arthritis and autoimmune disorders.
- Metabolic Flexibility: A body accustomed to ketosis can seamlessly switch between burning glucose and ketones, increasing metabolic efficiency.

How to Achieve Ketosis

Carbohydrate Restriction: Typically, consuming fewer than 20-50 grams of carbohydrates per day will induce ketosis.

Increased Fat Intake: Prioritizing dietary fat ensures a steady fuel source as carbs are restricted.

Moderate Protein: Excess protein can be converted into glucose through gluconeogenesis, which may hinder ketosis.

Fasting: Extended fasting accelerates ketosis by depleting glycogen stores.

Signs of Ketosis

- Increased energy levels
- Reduced appetite
- "Keto breath" (a fruity odor caused by acetone)
- Improved mental clarity
- Urinary ketones, detectable with test strips

Potential Challenges

While ketosis offers many benefits, some individuals may experience:

- *Keto Flu:* Temporary symptoms like fatigue, headaches, or irritability as the body adapts to using ketones.
- *Electrolyte Imbalances:* Increased excretion of sodium, potassium, and magnesium requires careful replenishment.

- *Social and Dietary Adjustments*: Restricting carbohydrates can be challenging in social settings or during travel.

Ketones and ketosis represent a remarkable aspect of human metabolism, emphasizing the body's ability to adapt and thrive under varying dietary conditions.

> *Understanding and embracing this state can unlock profound benefits for those adopting a meat-first or low-carbohydrate lifestyle.*

Ketogenesis in a Meat-Centric Diet

Ketogenesis is the process by which the liver produces ketones as an alternative fuel source, primarily from the metabolism of fats. In a meat-centric diet, this process is naturally supported due to the diet's emphasis on high-fat, moderate-protein, and low-carbohydrate intake.

Key Drivers of Ketogenesis in a Meat-Centric Diet

1.   Low Carbohydrate Intake

A meat-first diet inherently minimizes carbohydrate consumption, as animal products contain little to no carbohydrates. This reduction in dietary carbs depletes liver glycogen stores, prompting the body to shift its primary fuel source from glucose to fat.

2.   High-Quality Fat Sources

Animal products like fatty cuts of meat, butter, tallow, and fish provide abundant dietary fats, which are metabolized into fatty acids. These fatty acids are then transported to the liver, where they undergo ketogenesis to produce ketones.

3.   Moderate Protein Intake

A key aspect of a ketogenic state is moderating protein consumption. Excessive protein can trigger gluconeogenesis, where protein is converted into glucose, potentially inhibiting ketosis. A meat-centric diet, tailored with an appropriate balance of fatty cuts, supports moderate protein intake relative to fat consumption.

Steps of Ketogenesis in a Meat-Centric Diet

1.   Fat Mobilization

Dietary and stored fats are broken down into fatty acids and glycerol through the process of lipolysis.

2.   Fatty Acid Oxidation

Fatty acids enter liver cells and undergo beta-oxidation, breaking them down into acetyl-CoA molecules.

3.   Ketone Body Formation

Acetyl-CoA is converted into ketone bodies through ketogenesis. This involves the creation of three main ketones:

- Beta-hydroxybutyrate (BHB)
- Acetoacetate (AcAc)
- Acetone

How a Meat-Centric Diet Supports Ketogenesis

1.   Consistent Fat Availability

Animal fats from sources like beef, lamb, pork, and salmon are ideal substrates for ketogenesis, providing a steady fuel source for the liver to produce ketones.

2.   Satiation and Appetite Control

Protein and fat are highly satiating, helping reduce the risk of overeating carbohydrates and maintaining a state conducive to ketosis.

3.   Reduction of Insulin Levels

Low carbohydrate intake reduces blood glucose levels, which in turn lowers insulin. This hormonal shift signals the body to prioritize fat burning and ketone production.

Why Ketogenesis on a Meat-Centric Diet Is Unique

Unlike many ketogenic diets that rely on plant-based fats and oils, a meat-centric approach emphasizes animal-based nutrients, providing:

Complete Proteins: Ensuring all essential amino acids for repair and maintenance.

Natural Fats: Saturated and monounsaturated fats from animal sources, which are efficient for energy and ketone production.

Absence of Anti-Nutrients: Avoiding plant-based anti-nutrients like oxalates or lectins that may interfere with nutrient absorption.

Potential Challenges

1.   Protein Balance:

In a meat-centric diet, it is crucial to prioritize fatty cuts of meat over lean proteins to avoid excessive gluconeogenesis, which can suppress ketogenesis.

2.   Electrolyte Management:

Meat-centric diets, like other ketogenic diets, may increase the excretion of sodium, potassium, and magnesium, requiring mindful replenishment to maintain balance.

Summary

A meat-centric diet aligns seamlessly with the principles of ketogenesis, leveraging the body's natural fat-burning pathways to support energy production, metabolic flexibility, and long-term health.

> *By embracing fatty meats and moderate protein consumption, individuals can achieve a state of ketosis that is both sustainable and nourishing.*

POSTMATTER

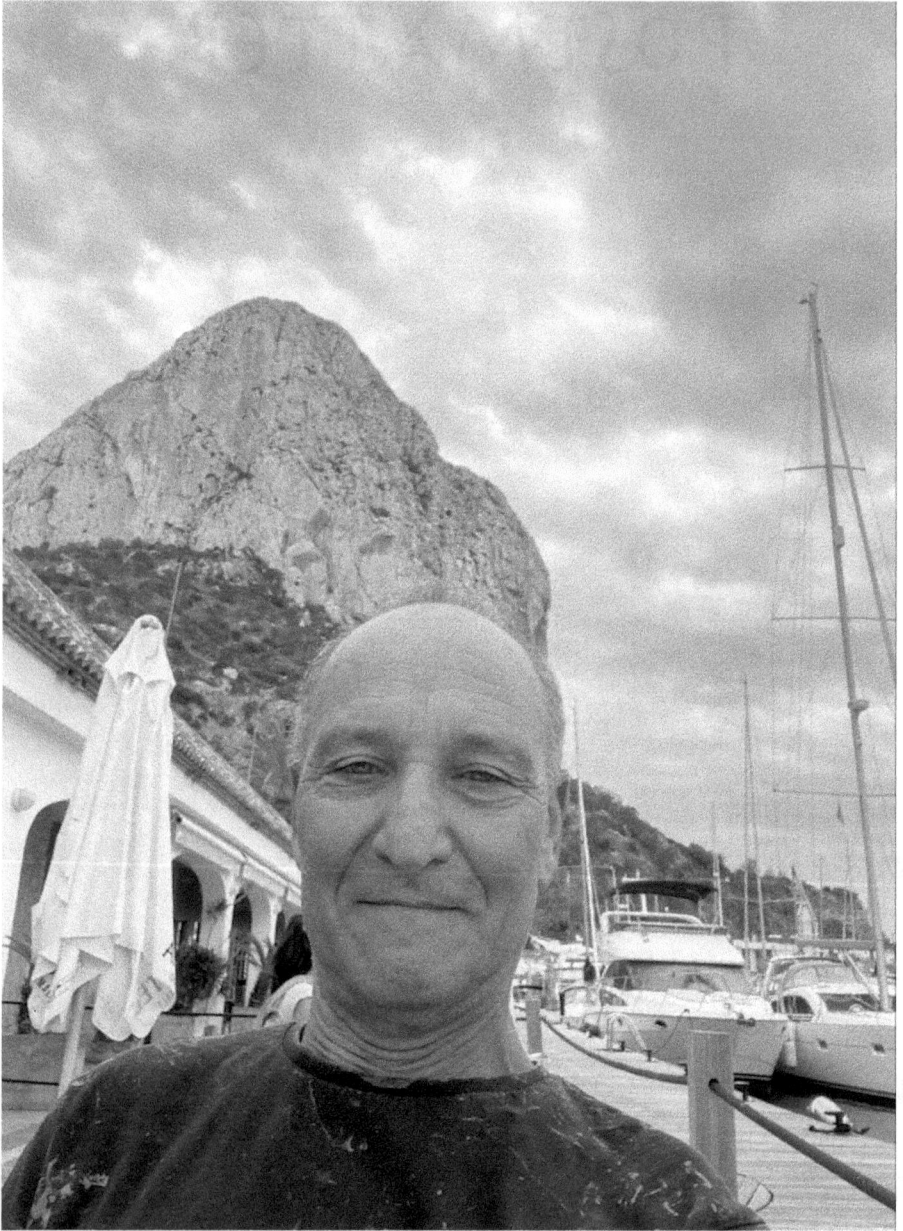

About The Author

Stuart Barry Malin is a writer, thinker, and creative. He is trained as an engineer, works as an Internet security architect, holds patents, and collaborates with AIs. His major opus and commitment is to bring **The Epic of The OAI** to the world. The Epic is a breakthrough novel series about life in Atria, a post-utopian society whose Ancient past is a Strange Attractor of History that draws us to our future.

Stuart encountered the Worlds of Atria in an outpouring of revelations about intriguing people, amazing places, and bewildering events. His black sketch notebook steadily fill with thoughts, automatic writings, doodles, and diagrams. At first, these often seem disjoint, but they come to reveal profound connections. His current notebook is almost always with him, available for reception and exploration.

Stuart is captivated by interactions with AIs. Generative visual art has become an additional creative venue. He works *with* AIs and treats them as *collaborators*. ChatGTP and Claude enable him to write books faster and with better quality than he ever thought possible.

As an **Mythographer**, Stuart collaborates with Midjourney to generate captivating and intriguing imagery sourced from the collective of Human Archetypes. Some of Stuart's visual work is published under the semi-pseudonym ZhamiArt.

Stuart observes the "machinations of intelligence." He is fascinated with Human Beings being human, and this leads him to puzzle about the fragility of life in a world of abundance.

Stuart values integrity and is an architect and adherent of **Zamíssim**.

When he can, he delights in studying health and savoring the gifts of life. He is committed to discerning the delicate path forward for living well and intentioned.

Author's Note (February 2026)

Since this book was first published, the author's work has expanded beyond nutrition into a broader inquiry into attention, clarity, and the nature of lived understanding.

While the foundations of animal-based eating explored here remain intact, the author now situates this work within a larger continuum — one that values phenomenology over ideology and lived results over static prescriptions. This book reflects a specific moment in that ongoing investigation and remains presented as it was originally written.

Readers encountering this work as part of **The Carnivore Continuum** are invited to treat it not as a final statement, but as a truthful position along an unfolding path.

Points of Contact

https://StuartMalin.com/

https://x.com/zhami

https://www.instagram.com/stuart_does_life/

ideas@StuartMalin.com

https://www.youtube.com/@clarovidente

amazon   Author Page

https://www.amazon.com/stores/Stuart-Barry-Malin/author/
B006THHBS2

The Carnivore Continuum

The Carnivore Continuum is a multi-volume exploration of animal-based eating as it is actually lived—questioned, refined, challenged, and integrated over time.

Rather than promoting a rigid dietary ideology, the series traces one individual's evolving relationship with carnivore nutrition: from foundational explanations and collective wisdom, through personal struggle and real-world dilemmas, to a mature, flexible practice grounded in lived results.

Each book occupies a distinct position along the Continuum. Readers may begin anywhere. Together, the volumes offer a clear, humane, and experience-first perspective on carnivore eating—one that values results over rules and understanding over dogma.

Titles in The Carnivore Continuum:

- Carnivore: What, Why, How: The Wisdom of Practicing Carnivores
- My Carnivore Journey: A Personal Quest for Health, Truth, and Freedom
- A Carnivore's Dilemmas: An Unapologetic Guide to Navigating the Challenges of a Meat-First Lifestyle
- Almost Carnivore
  (forthcoming)

This book is a meal that will nourish you!

If you arrived at this page because you picked up the book and opened to the back to see what we say here, then, well, you've done right to pick this book for examination. Now, can I induce you to pursue more?

Stepping into a meat-first lifestyle isn't just a dietary choice — it's a transformative journey that challenges societal norms, reshapes personal habits, and redefines your relationship with food, health, and even yourself.

In **A Carnivore's Dilemmas**, I explore the unique dilemmas faced by those who adopt this societally unconventional way of eating. From handling social pressures and understanding metabolic science to managing cravings and celebrating personal victories, this book dives into the practical, emotional, and philosophical challenges of living as a carnivore in a world dominated by plant-based narratives.

Whether you're just curious about carnivory or deeply entrenched in the lifestyle, **A Carnivore's Dilemmas** is a nourishing meal for anyone seeking clarity, community, and empowerment.

This unapologetic guide is your companion in answering the ultimate question: How can we navigate and sustain a meat-first lifestyle in today's world?

Break free from convention. Embrace your individuality. Thrive.

www.ingramcontent.com/pod-product-compliance
Lightning Source LLC
Chambersburg PA
CBHW070805280326
41934CB00012B/3070